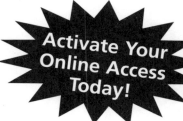

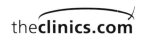

CARDIOLOGY CLINICS

Patent Foramen Ovale

GUEST EDITORS
Edward A. Gill, Jr, MD
John D. Carroll, MD

CONSULTING EDITOR
Michael H. Crawford, MD

February 2005 • Volume 23 • Number 1

SAUNDERS

An Imprint of Elsevier, Inc.
PHILADELPHIA   LONDON   TORONTO   MONTREAL   SYDNEY   TOKYO

W.B. SAUNDERS COMPANY
A Division of Elsevier Inc.

The Curtis Center • Independence Square West • Philadelphia, Pennsylvania 19106

http://www.theclinics.com

CARDIOLOGY CLINICS
February 2005
Editor: Karen Sorensen

Volume 23, Number 1
ISSN 0733-8651
ISBN 1-4160-2698-3

Reprints. For copies of 100 or more, of articles in this publication, please contact the Commercial Reprints Department, Elsevier Inc., 360 Park Avenue South, New York, New York 10010-1710. Tel. (212) 633-3813 Fax: (212) 462-1935 email: reprints@elsevier.com

The ideas and opinions expressed in *Cardiology Clinics* do not necessarily reflect those of the Publisher. The Publisher does not assume any responsibility for any injury and/or damage to persons or property arising out of or related to any use of the material contained in this periodical. The reader is advised to check the appropriate medical literature and the product information currently provided by the manufacturer of each drug to be administered to verify the dosage, the method and duration of administration, or contraindications. It is the responsibility of the treating physician or other health care professional, relying on independent experience and knowledge of the patient, to determine drug dosages and the best treatment for the patient. Mention of any product in this issue should not be construed as endorsement by the contributors, editors, or the Publisher of the product or manufacturers' claims.

Cardiology Clinics (ISSN 0733-8651) is published quarterly by W.B. Saunders Company; Corporate and editorial Offices: The Curtis Center, Independence Square West, Philadelphia, PA 19106-3399. Accounting and circulation offices: 6277 Sea Harbor Drive, Orlando, FL 32887-4800. Periodicals postage paid at Orlando, FL 32862, and additional mailing offices. Subscription prices are $170.00 per year for US individuals, $266.00 per year for US institutions, $85.00 per year for US students and residents, $210.00 per year for Canadian individuals, $323.00 per year for Canadian institutions, $230.00 per year for international individuals, $323.00 per year for international institutions and $115.00 per year for Canadian and foreign students/residents. To receive student/resident rate, orders must be accompanied by name of affiliated institution, data of term, and the *signature* of program/residency coordinator on institution letterhead. Orders will be billed at individual rate until proof of status is received. Foreign air speed delivery is included in all *Clinics* subscription prices. All prices are subject to change without notice. POSTMASTER: Send address changes to *Cardiology Clinics*, W.B. Saunders Company, Periodicals Fulfillment, Orlando, FL 32887-4800. **Customer Service: 1-800-654-2452 (US). From outside of the US, call 1-407-345-1000.**

Cardiology Clinics is also published in Spanish by McGraw-Hill Interamericana Editores S. A., P.O. Box 5-237, 06500, Mexico D. F., Mexico; in Portuguese by Reichmann and Alfonso Editores Rio de Janeiro, Brazil; and in Greek by Dimitrios P. Lagos, 8 Pondon Street, GR115-28 Ilissia, Greece.

Cardiology Clinics is covered in *Index Medicus, Excerpta Medica, The Cumulative Index to Nursing and Allied Health Literature* (INAHL).

CONSULTING EDITOR

MICHAEL H. CRAWFORD, MD, Professor, Department of Medicine, University of California Medical School; and Chief of Clinical Cardiology, Division of Cardiology, University of California, San Francisco, San Francisco, California

GUEST EDITORS

EDWARD A. GILL, Jr, MD, Associate Professor, Division of Cardiology, Department of Medicine, University of Washington School of Medicine, Seattle; and Director, Echocardiography Division, Harborview Medical Center, Seattle, Washington

JOHN D. CARROLL, MD, Professor, Department of Medicine; and Director, Interventional Cardiology Section, Cardiovascular Division, University of Colorado Health Sciences Center, Denver, Colorado

CONTRIBUTORS

RACHEL DONAHUE BEDA, MD, Department of Medicine, University of Washington School of Medicine, Seattle, Washington

MARK BOUCEK, MD, Professor, Department of Pediatrics, University of Colorado Health Sciences Center, Denver, Colorado; and Chief, Department of Cardiology, Joe DiMaggio Children's Hospital, Hollywood, Florida

JOHN D. CARROLL, MD, Professor, Department of Medicine; and Director, Interventional Cardiology Section, Cardiovascular Division, University of Colorado Health Sciences Center, Denver, Colorado

GRACE PEI-WEN CHEN, MD, Division of Cardiology, Department of Medicine, University of Washington School of Medicine, Seattle, Washington

STEVEN C. CRAMER, MD, Assistant Professor, Department of Neurology, University of California, Irvine Medical Center, University of California Irvine, Orange, California

STEPHEN DODGE, MD, Interventional Cardiology Section, Cardiovascular Division, Health Sciences Center, University of Colorado, Denver, Colorado

PETER GERMONPRÉ, MD, Medical Director, Centre for Hyperbaric Oxygen Therapy, Military Hospital Brussels, Brussels, Belgium

EDWARD A. GILL, Jr, MD, Associate Professor, Division of Cardiology, Department of Medicine, University of Washington School of Medicine, Seattle; and Director, Echocardiography Division, Harborview Medical Center, Seattle, Washington

STEVEN L. GOLDBERG, MD, Associate Professor, Division of Cardiology, Department of Medicine, University of Washington Medical School, Seattle; and Acting Director, Cardiac Catheterization Laboratory, Seattle, Washington

BERTRON M. GROVES, MD, Professor, Departments of Medicine and Radiology, Interventional Cardiology Section, Cardiovascular Division, University of Colorado Health Sciences Center, Denver, Colorado

KATHRYN L. HASSELL, MD, Associate Professor, Division of Hematology, Department of Medicine, University of Colorado Health Sciences Center, Denver, Colorado

SAMIR R. KAPADIA, MD, Cleveland Clinic Foundation, Cleveland, Ohio

ROBERT A. QUAIFE, MD, Associate Professor, Division of Cardiology, Department of Medicine, University of Colorado Health Sciences Center, Denver, Colorado

CONTENTS

FORTHCOMING ISSUES

RECENT ISSUES

ELSEVIER
SAUNDERS

Cardiol Clin 23 (2005) ix

CARDIOLOGY
CLINICS

Foreword

Patent Foramen Ovale

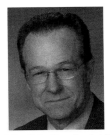

Michael H. Crawford, MD
Consulting Editor

This issue of the *Cardiology Clinics* focuses on the problem of patent foramen ovale (PFO). Formerly regarded as an anatomic variant often found at autopsy and of little or no consequence, PFO is now the subject of intense scrutiny. The advent of echocardiography with agitated saline contrast has lead to increased premortem diagnosis of this condition. Clinical correlation studies with cerebral vascular accidents, headaches, and other conditions have lead to the hypothesis that adverse events could be due to this anomaly. However, early on in our recognition of this condition, the only effective therapy was surgical closure. Thus, medical therapy was tried, such as oral anticoagulation in patients with PFO and cryptogenic stroke, reserving surgery for drug therapy–resistant patients with recurrent events. This all changed with the development of the percutaneous closure device. Now PFOs can be closed with low risk and very short recovery times using these new devices. This development has broadened the application of these devices and lead to new thinking about the etiology of the blood clots that travel through this potential shunt.

I was delighted when Dr. Gill from the University of Washington in Seattle and Dr. Carroll from the University of Colorado in Denver agreed to compile this issue. Dr. Gill is an echocardiographer and Dr. Carroll is an interventional cardiologist—an ideal team to lead such an effort, considering echocardiography plays such a large role in this interventional technique. They have assembled an outstanding group of authors who cover every aspect of this emerging technology and its applications. This topic has achieved sufficient maturity that all who care for patients need to be knowledgeable about it. This issue admirably achieves that goal.

Michael H. Crawford, MD
Division of Cardiology
University of California
505 Parnassus Avenue, Box 0124
San Francisco, CA 94143-0124, USA

E-mail address: crawfordm@medicine.ucsf.edu

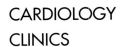
CARDIOLOGY
CLINICS

Cardiol Clin 23 (2005) xi–xii

Preface

Patent Foramen Ovale: No Longer an Innocent Remnant of Fetal Circulation

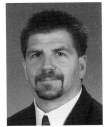 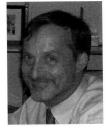

Edward A. Gill, Jr, MD   John D. Carroll, MD
Guest Editors

Approximately 25% of the general population has a patent foramen ovale (PFO); that percentage is higher in those younger than 35 years of age and less in those older. The absolute number varies depending both on the series and on the method used to diagnose the PFO and whether it is an autopsy series. In the vast majority of people with PFO, there is absolutely no consequence to this anatomic variant of normal. However, in some the PFO may be the pathway through which thrombotic emboli, air emboli, desaturated blood, and vasoactive substances are shunted and enter the left atrium without traversing the pulmonary circulation. Paradoxical emboli clearly play a role in the development of stroke. In other patients, the PFO has a role in the pathophysiology of hypoxia. Clearly however, the major clinical problem has been the striking association of PFO with stroke in young and middle-aged people. Hence the challenge in both daily practice and in the design and conduct of clinical trials is to determine which patients with PFO are at risk for either initial or recurrent stroke and then to try to prevent it.

While it has become clear that some PFOs should be closed, it is just as clear that not all PFOs should be closed as a prophylaxis against stroke. For those individuals who have experienced recurrent cryptogenic stroke despite optimal medical therapy and PFO, the advice is clear: PFO closure should be strongly considered, either surgically, or more recently, by percutaneous methods. For those individuals with first-time stroke, no other clear cause (ie, cryptogenic), and PFO, the choice of treatment is much less clear. Our goal in this issue of the *Cardiology Clinics* is to shed some light on the latter group of patients; however, complete certainty with regard to treatment will not be within reach until the unveiling of studies that truly randomize patients to closure versus an accepted medical regimen. It is also disconcerting that even experts in the field cannot agree on the best medical regimen.

Next, with regard to percutaneous methods, the state-of-the-art approach to this method of closure of PFO will be discussed in some detail. The procedure involves skill sets not common in the adult interventional cardiology community. The procedure has been developed and refined through collaboration between pediatric and adult interventional cardiologists. The procedure should be performed with a very small risk of complication and a high degree of successful and complete closure of the PFO.

There are intriguing hematologic associations with stroke and PFO and indeed, PFO may be only a necessary but not sufficient reason for stroke in these patients. Hypercoagulable diseases and other measureable tendencies toward intravascular thrombus formation have been discovered in the past few decades. The hematologist has become an important part of the professional team evaluating individual patients and designing clinical trials to better understand the pathophysiology of thromboembolic clinical syndromes such as PFO-associated stroke.

Anatomic variations and the "tunneling" affect of the PFO may also be a nidus for thrombus development. The role of echocardiography is central in studying PFO, especially transesophageal and intracardiac echocardiography, because it can characterize PFO physiology, the septum secundum and primum, and associated structures such as the Eustachian valve and Chiari network. Image guidance of percutaneous implantation of PFO closure devices is typically by a combination of fluoroscopy and ultrasound.

Finally, PFO has relevance in other medical conditions, particularly migraine headache,

platnypnea-orthodeoxia, and the decompression sickness of divers. We suspect that readers will be enticed by the discussion of these rather unique situations.

Edward A. Gill, Jr, MD
Department of Medicine
Division of Cardiology
Harborview Medical Center
325 Ninth Avenue
Seattle, WA 98104, USA

E-mail address: eagill@u.washington.edu

John D. Carroll, MD
Department of Interventional Cardiology
University of Colorado Health Sciences Center
4200 E. Ninth Avenue
Denver, CO 80262, USA

E-mail address: john.carroll@uchsc.edu

ELSEVIER
SAUNDERS

Cardiol Clin 23 (2005) 1–6

CARDIOLOGY
CLINICS

Definitions and Pathophysiology of the Patent Foramen Ovale: Broad Overview

Edward A. Gill, Jr, MD[a,b,*]

[a]Division of Cardiology, Department of Medicine, University of Washington, 1959 Pacific Avenue NE,
Seattle, WA 98195, USA
[b]Harborview Medical Center, 325 Ninth Avenue, Seattle, WA 98104, USA

The fossa ovalis is the indentation on the right atrial side of the interatrial septum that is present when a foramen ovale is closed. This is the semantic distinction between the fossa ovalis and patent foramen ovale (PFO) [1]. Whether the foramen ovale is open (PFO) or closed (fossa ovalis), the location is directly adjacent to the triangle of Koch. The anterior margin of the coronary sinus, the tricuspid annulus, and the tendon of Todaro define the triangle of Koch (Fig. 1). The foramen ovale or opening on the right atrial side is just superior and anterior to the triangle of Koch [2]. The ostium secundum, the opening of the PFO on the left atrial side, is more superior yet. There is a tunnel, however short, from the foramen ovale on the right side of the atrium to the opening of the ostium secundum on the left side. This tunnel takes a superior track. The length of the tunnel is of particular importance for the percutaneous closure procedure [3]. When a long tunnel is present, consideration must be given to performing a trans-septal puncture through the center of the tunnel and placing the closure device across the newly created hole [3]. This technique avoids malpositioning of the device because of a long tunnel.

Definition of patent foramen ovale

From an anatomic perspective, the PFO is a communication between the atria that begins at the area of the fossa ovalis on the right atrial side and traverses to the ostium secundum on the left side. The flow through the foramen ovale depends on the flap of tissue formed by the septum primum remaining open following embryonic development (Figs. 2 and 3). In fetal life, normal blood flow passes from the right atrium to the left atrium through the PFO, bypassing the nonfunctioning lungs (Fig. 4). With the first breath of a newborn, the PFO closes as pressure in the left atrium rises to a level higher than right atrial pressure. This difference in pressure causes the septum primum (on the left side of the interatrial septum) to be compressed into the septum secundum (on the right side of the interatrial septum), resulting in closure of the PFO (Fig. 5). Hence, the septum primum is essentially a valve structure that normally should be closed because of higher pressure in the left atrium than in the right atrium. A PFO is different from an atrial septal defect. The former results from lack of fusion of the septum primum and septum secundum; the latter results from a failure in the formation of the interatrial septum. The normal sequence is for the septum primum and septum secundum to fuse and create an intact interatrial septum that is impermeable to the passage of red blood cells and certainly is impermeable to clots. This fusion occurs in most individuals by 2 years of age. Echocardiographic and autopsy studies, however, have shown that fusion is never completely accomplished in approximately 25% of the

* Division of Harborview Electrocardiography, Department of Medicine, University of Washington School of Medicine, 1959 Pacific Avenue NE, Box 35948, Seattle, WA 98195.
    E-mail address: eagill@u.washington.edu

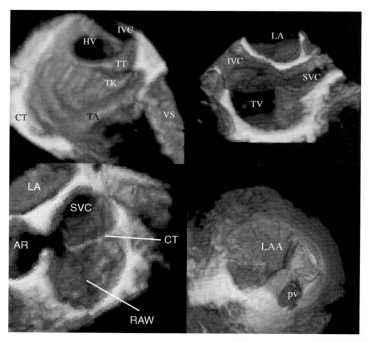

Fig. 1. The triangle of Koch. Important landmarks within the right atrium are shown. The triangle of Koch is defined by the coronary sinus, tricuspid annulus, and the tendon of Todaro. The anatomy of the structures surrounding the fossa ovalis is important in determining a diagnosis of patent foramen ovale therapeutically with regard to percutaneous closure of the defect. AR, aortic root; CT, crista terminalis; HV, hepatic vein; IVC, inferior vena cava; LAA, left atrial appendage; PV, pulmonary valve; RAW, right atrial wall; SVC, superior vena cava; TA, tricuspid annulus; TK, triangle of Koch; TT, tendon of Todaro; TV, tricuspid annulus; VS, ventricular septum. (Courtesy of V.L. Sorrell, MD, Tuscon, AZ.)

population. The percentage decreases with age from roughly 35% before age 30 years to roughly 22% at 90 years [1]. In addition, there is a clear continuum for degree of closure with some PFOs patent only to a probe at the time of autopsy. On the other end of the spectrum there are PFOs that are quite widely patent and allow a significant amount of shunting even at rest or without any maneuvers.

By echocardiography, the definition of a PFO is a communication between the atria that allows right-to-left shunting as detected by either color or spectral Doppler or by an agitated saline contrast study. As detailed, in article by Gill and Quaife that discusses the echocardiographic evaluation of PFO, the shunt may not be unveiled until the patient performs the Valsalva maneuver or coughs. In some cases, the echocardiographic definition is clouded because foramen ovale connections allow bidirectional or left-to-right shunting as well as right-to-left shunting, particularly when the fora- men ovale has fenestrations or has been stretched, as in heart failure, (Fig. 6). In the case of stretching

in heart failure, a more correct description is stretching of the septum primum that results in a larger ostium secundum and essentially in an interatrial communication that is present through- out the cardiac cycle. From an echocardiographic view, particularly a transthoracic echo view, this finding may be indistinguishable from an atrial septal defect and can be identified correctly only by considering the clinical setting in which it occurs and by making a concerted effort to identify the septum primum anatomically. This identification will probably be possible only by means of trans- esophageal echo study.

Pathophysiology of a foramen ovale

In most cases the physiologic significance of a PFO is limited to the theoretical possibility of a paradoxicalal embolus that could cause a stroke. Paradoxicalal embolus through a PFO was first described in 1877 [4]. Stroke and PFO is the topic of another article in this volume. To summarize

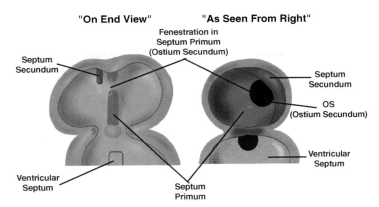

Fig. 2. The initial formation of the interatrial septum is shown with the initial development of the septum primum on the left side of the interatrial septum. Fenestrations in the septum primum form the basis of the opening for the ostium secundum which will be the opening of the foramen ovale on the left side. Note that at the same time, the septum secundum is developing on the right side of the interatrial septum. (*Modified from* CathSAP, American College of Cardiology Foundation.)

briefly, a PFO is believed to be important in the pathophysiology of cryptogenic stroke, particularly in patients younger than 55 years of age.

There is evidence that some individuals develop right-to-left shunting during exercise, potentially leading to hypoxia [5]. In certain conditions, the presence of a PFO can lead to a dramatic degree of right-to-left shunting, sufficient to cause hypoxia. Examples of such conditions include severe pulmonary hypertension with right atrial hypertension and tricuspid stenosis. Of particular significance is a prosthetic valve in the tricuspid position. Because the orifice area of a prosthetic valve is not as large as that of the native valve, particularly the tricuspid valve, a significant

gradient is present across the valve. Finally, in left-sided heart failure, mitral stenosis, or any condition leading to left atrial enlargement, the left atrium, and in particular the ostium secundum, becomes stretched, often leading to significant left-to-right shunting (see Fig. 6). Mitral stenosis and a stretched PFO is likely to be misdiagnosed by echocardiography as syndrome of Luttembacher (ie, mitral stenosis and an atrial septal defect).

Other conditions that seem to be particularly worsened in the setting of a PFO include migraine headaches and decompression sickness in divers. In fact, in a group of seven divers, two cases of marked desaturation with treadmill exercise were

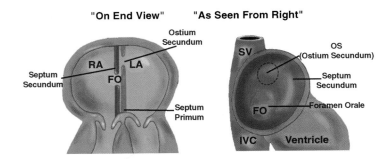

Fig. 3. At this stage of development, the septum secundum has formed and a fenestration within this septum is the opening for the foramen ovale. Note that blood flows from the foramen ovale superior and anterior to then pass through the ostium secundum. Note that the distance between the foramen ovale on the right and the ostium secundum on the left will form the basis of a 'tunnel' that will be discussed in other sections with regard to challenges it presents for closing a patent foramen ovale. (*Modified from* CathSAP, American College of Cardiology Foundation.)

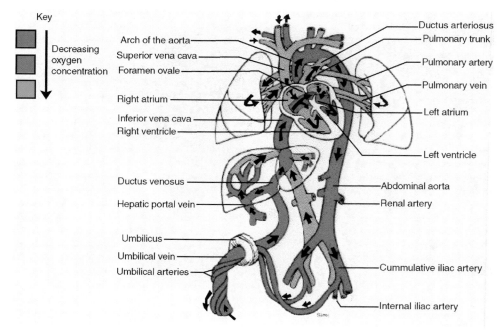

Fig. 4. Fetal circulation. This diagram outlines the course of flow from the inferior vena cava to the right atrium and ultimately through the patent foramen ovale. Flow from the inferior vena cava flow is preferentially directed at the patent foramen ovale by the Eustachian valve, and, if present, the Chiari network, a stringlike network that is an extension of the Eustachian valve.

noted; one case was as low as 80% [6]. Further, there seems to be an increased risk of ischemic stroke in patients with migraines and a PFO [7–9].

In the absence of certain conditions or activities, the PFO is an insignificant structure unless a thrombus forms somewhere in the venous circulation and becomes lodged or crosses the PFO, causing a paradoxical embolus. Such an event is most likely to result in a stroke but can also manifest as a peripheral artery embolus or an

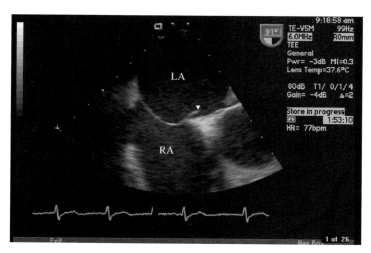

Fig. 5. Transesophageal echocardiogram of a prominent septum primum in a patient with a patent foramen ovale (*arrowhead*). Note the rather dramatic bowing of the interatrial septum from left to right. LA, left atrium; RA, right atrium.

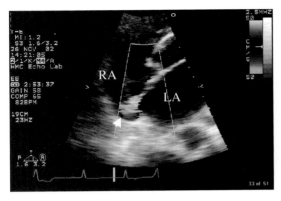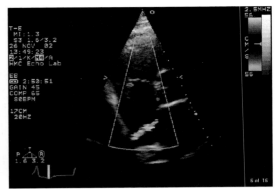

Fig. 6. Two similar views of a stretched patent foramen ovale with left-to-right shunting in a patient with a dilated left atrium resulting from heart failure. The views are parasternal short-axis views by transthoracic echo showing flow from the left atrium to the right atrium.

embolus to an organ such as the kidneys or spleen that causes an infarct. Organ infarcts are likely to be silent unless they are quite large.

There is now mounting evidence that stroke may be more likely to develop in patients who have a PFO if they also have an underlying hypercoagulable state or thrombophilia. Of the prothrombotic states, Factor V Leiden and the prothrombin gene mutations may prove to carry notably increased risk for stroke. These factors are discussed further in another article in this issue.

Size of the patent foramen ovale and relationship of size to physiologic importance

According to one autopsy study, the size of a PFO ranges from 1 to 19 mm with a mean diameter of 4.9 mm [1]. The size of a PFO has been shown to correlate with the risk of stroke in a number of studies using different methods to measure the size of the PFO [10–15]. So far, in prospective studies evaluating patients with known stroke and recurrent events, the size of the defect has not emerged as an important variable for recurrence [16].

Mechanisms for normal closure of the patent foramen ovale and the potential role of genetics in lack of closure

The reason the foramen ovale does not close in roughly 25% of individuals is not known. Some rare families have transmission of atrial septal defect in an autosomal dominant pattern. One

study has suggested that PFO can also be a familial trait [17]. In this study, siblings of women with PFO were more likely to have PFO than siblings of women without PFO. Whether a familial pattern of stroke and PFO exists remains to be elucidated.

References

[1] Hagen PT, Scholz DG, Edwards WD. Incidence and size of patent foramen ovale during the first 10 decades of life: an autopsy study of 965 normal hearts. Mayo Clin Proc 1984;59:17–20.

[2] Anderson RH, Brown NA, Webb S. Development and structure of the atrial septum. Heart 2002;88:104–10.

[3] McMahon CJ, El Said HG, Mullins CE. Use of the transseptal puncture in transcatheter closure of long tunnel-type patent foramen ovale. Heart 2002;88:E3.

[4] Mas JL. Patent foramen ovale, stroke and paradoxicalal embolism. Cerebrovasc Dis 1991;1:181–3.

[5] Wilmhurst P, Nightingale S. Relationship between migraine and cardiac and pulmonary right-to-left shunts. Clin Sci 2001;100:215–20.

[6] Wilmhurts PT, Treacher DF, Crowther A, et al. Effects of a patent foramen ovale on arterial saturation during exercise and on cardiovascular responses to deep breathing, Valsalva maneuvre, and passive tilt: relation to history of decompression illness in divers. Br Heart J 1994;71:229–31.

[7] Wilmhurst PT, Nightingale, Walsh KP, et al. Effect on migraine of closure of cardiac right-to-left shunts to prevent recurrence of decompression illness or stroke or for haemodynamic reasons. Lancet 2000;356:1648–51.

[8] Crassard I, Conard J, Bousser M-G. Migraine and haemostatsis. Cephalagia 2001;21:630–6.

[9] Tzourio C, Kittner SJ, Bousser M-G, et al. Migraine and stroke in young women. Cephalagia 2000;20: 190–9.

[10] Homma S, DiTullio MR, Sacco RL, et al. Characteristics of patent foramen ovale associated with cryptogenic stroke. A biplane transesophageal echocardiographic study. Stroke 1994;25:582–6.

[11] Job FP, Ringelstein B, Grafen Y, et al. Comparison of transcranial contrast Doppler sonography and transesophageal contrast echocardiography for the detection of patent foramen ovale in young stroke patients. Am J Cardiol 1994;74:381–4.

[12] Steiner MM, Di Tullio MR, Rundek T, et al. Patent foramen ovale size and embolic brain imaging findings among patients with ischemic stroke. Stroke 1998;29:944–8.

[13] Schuchlenz HW, Weihs W, Beitzke A, et al. Transesophageal echocardiography for quantifying size of patent foramen ovale in patients with cryptogenic cerebrovascular events. Stroke 2002;33:293–6.

[14] Kerut EK, Norfleet WT, Plotnick GD, et al. Patent foramen ovale: a review of associated conditions and the impact of physiologic size. J Am Coll Cardiol 2001;38:613–23.

[15] Kerr AJ, Buck T, Chia K, et al. Transmitral Doppler: a new transthoracic contrast method for patent foramen ovale detection and quantification. J Am Coll Cardiol 2000;35:1959–66.

[16] Homma S, Sacco RL, Di Tullio MR, et al. Effect of medical treatment in stroke patients with patent foramen ovale: patent foramen ovale in the Cryptogenic Stroke Study. Circulation 2002;105: 2625–31.

[17] Arquizan C, Coste J, Touboul P-J, et al. Is patent foramen ovale a family trait. A transcranial Doppler sonographic study. Stroke 2001;32:1563–6.

ELSEVIER
SAUNDERS

CARDIOLOGY
CLINICS

Cardiol Clin 23 (2005) 7–11

Patent Foramen Ovale and its Relationship to Stroke

Steven C. Cramer, MD

*Department of Neurology, University of California, Irvine Medical Center, University of California, Irvine,
101 The City Drive South, Orange, CA 92868-4280, USA*

Stroke is a major medical problem. It remains the leading cause of adult disability and is the third leading cause of death in the United States and in many other countries, with an estimated annual cost in the United States exceeding $40 billion [1]. More than 700,000 new strokes are diagnosed each year in the United States [2]. Approximately 4.5 million stroke survivors are currently alive in the United States [3]. The median survival after a stroke is 7 years, during which time patients are at a greater risk for stroke recurrence than the general population.

The term "stroke" refers to an interruption of the blood supply to the brain, resulting in brain injury and often accompanied by new clinical deficits. About 85% of strokes are ischemic, and 15% are hemorrhagic. An ischemic stroke can be caused by many different pathophysiologic processes. Several studies suggest that the cause of ischemic strokes is a large-artery process such as internal carotid artery narrowing in 20% to 25% of patients, a small-artery process such as those that produce a lacune in 20% of patients, and a cardioembolic process such as atrial fibrillation in 20% to 25% of patients. These studies also suggest that no cause for a stroke can be found in 30% to 40% of patients [4–9]. When patients younger than 55 years of age were studied, no cause for stroke was apparent in 64% of patients [10]. Stroke of undetermined pathogenesis has been referred to as "cryptogenic stroke" [11].

Cryptogenic stroke probably represents a number of different disease processes. Nevertheless, a large percentage of patients with a cryptogenic stroke share certain clinical features. Chief among these is an increased prevalence of a patent foramen ovale (PFO) [12].

Anatomic closure of the foramen ovale normally follows functional closure after birth, but an interatrial communication remains patent in a percentage of the normal population. An autopsy study by Thompson and Evans [13] found that 6% of subjects had a PFO that was pencil patent (>5 mm diameter), and 29% of subjects had a PFO that was probe patent (2–5 mm in diameter). More recently, Hagen et al [14] found that across all subjects at autopsy, 27.3% of subjects had a PFO, with mean diameter of 5 mm. This study also found that subjects younger than age 30 years had a higher prevalence of PFO, 34.3%, suggesting that the impact of disease processes related to a PFO may be greater in younger patients. Echocardiographic studies have varied in their estimates of PFO prevalence among healthy subjects, but results are generally lower than values found in autopsy studies, suggesting this noninvasive method has less sensitivity than direct anatomic inspection for identifying PFO. The prevalence of PFO found in most echocardiography studies of normal subjects has been between 10% [15] and 22% [16].

A PFO has been found to be present more often in patients with cryptogenic stroke than in patients with stroke of determined origin [10,15–25] or in normal controls [10,15,16,19,26–28]. A PFO with concomitant atrial septal aneurysm is also found more often in patients with cryptogenic stroke, particularly younger patients [12]. This dual diagnosis may have a greater association with stroke recurrence than either diagnosis alone [29].

Defining the prevalence of PFO is made difficult by the variability in diagnostic sensitivity of current noninvasive methods. Transesophageal

---

E-mail address: scramer@uci.edu

0733-8651/05/$ - see front matter © 2005 Elsevier Inc. All rights reserved.
doi:10.1016/j.ccl.2004.10.006

echocardiography (TEE) may be as much as two times more sensitive than transthoracic echocardiography for diagnosing a PFO [16,30]. (See, however, Ha et al, 2001 [31]) Transcranial Doppler has sensitivity that approaches that of TEE [20,32,33] but has decreased specificity. Although transcranial Doppler provides less information than echocardiography concerning cardiac structure, transcranial Doppler may be more sensitive to extracardiac right-to-left shunts. The choice of vein used to introduce echo contrast influences diagnostic sensitivity. Blood entering through the inferior vena cava is directed more toward the interatrial septum region where a PFO is found, as compared with blood entering the right atrium through the superior vena cava, Thus, studies have found that diagnostic sensitivity for a PFO is increased by 2.5-fold when agitated saline contrast is injected through the femoral vein rather than the antecubital vein [34,35].

The consistent observation that cryptogenic stroke is associated with an increased prevalence of PFO suggests that, in some of these patients, the PFO is a source or a conduit for thrombi embolizing to the brain. Other clinical characteristics commonly found in patients with cryptogenic stroke support this hypothesis. First, the topography of cerebral infarct in patients with cryptogenic stroke and PFO often suggests an embolic mechanism [4,24]. Second, PFO size is greater in patients with cryptogenic stroke than in with normal subjects or patients with stroke of determined origin [21,22,24–26,36], although PFO size may not influence stroke recurrence rates [25] (see also Kerut [37]). Third, the prevalence of PFO patency at rest (ie, without induction of a Valsalva-related pressure gradient) may be greater in patients with stroke than in control subjects [28].

A fourth line of evidence that may link PFO with pathophysiology of cryptogenic stroke is a significant prevalence of lower extremity deep venous thrombosis (DVT) in this patient population. Among patients with PFO and stroke or transient ischemic attack (TIA) of any cause, the prevalence of DVT has ranged from 6% [38] to 9.5% [30]. Another study reported a rate of 54% but had a relatively high representation of late DVT and stroke caused by atrial fibrillation [39]. Among patients with PFO and cryptogenic stroke/TIA, prevalences of 7% [23], 13% [40], 31% [41], and 27% [42] have been reported. Most studies addressing this point have been limited by evaluation of only a subset, rather than a consecutive cohort, of patients. Another frequent

limitation has been the absence of an appropriate control group, an important concern given the substantial increase in DVT prevalence that is found after stroke [43]. Direct evidence for increased frequency of DVT among patients with cryptogenic stroke and PFO is therefore limited. The Paradoxical Embolism from Large Veins in Ischemic Stroke (PELVIS) study addressed this issue. In the 5 center PELVIS study, patients 18 to 60 years of age received an MRI venogram (MRV) of the pelvis within 72 hours of new symptom onset. Compared with patients whose stroke was of determined origin (n = 49), patients with cryptogenic stroke (n = 46) were significantly younger, had a higher prevalence of PFO (61% versus 19%), and had less atherosclerosis risk factors. Also, cryptogenic patients had more MRV scans with a high probability for pelvic DVT (20%) than patients with stroke of determined origin (4%, P < 0.03), suggesting that paradoxical embolus from the pelvic veins may be the cause of stroke in a subset of patients classified as having cryptogenic stroke [44].

Consistent and thorough evaluation of the venous system after stroke may be important to clarify the role of PFO in the genesis of cryptogenic stroke. One issue that may be of particular importance is evaluation of calf veins. Emboli from calf vein thrombi tend to be small and asymptomatic on reaching the lung [45,46], but such emboli might be of substantially greater clinical significance upon reaching the cerebral circulation [11]. Study of the pelvic veins may also be important in the context of PFO-related stroke. In autopsy studies of patients with a paradoxical embolism, the pelvic veins were the only source of thromboemboli in 22% of patients [47,48]. A consecutive study of 769 MRI venograms found that 20% of the 167 DVT identified were isolated to the pelvic veins [49]. Pelvic DVT have been described in patients with cryptogenic pulmonary embolism [50–52] and in patients with cryptogenic stroke with PFO [41,42,53]. A patient diagnosed with paradoxical embolism caused by isolated pelvic DVT is presented in Fig. 1.

Even as the pathophysiology of cryptogenic stroke continues to be studied, clinicians have recognized that medical therapy in patients with a cryptogenic stroke may be associated with an important stroke recurrence rate, the precise value of which remains unclear. In patients with cryptogenic stroke/TIA, annual rates of recurrence have reported as 16% [54], 5.4% [28], 3.4% [55], and 3.8% (84% were cryptogenic in this study)

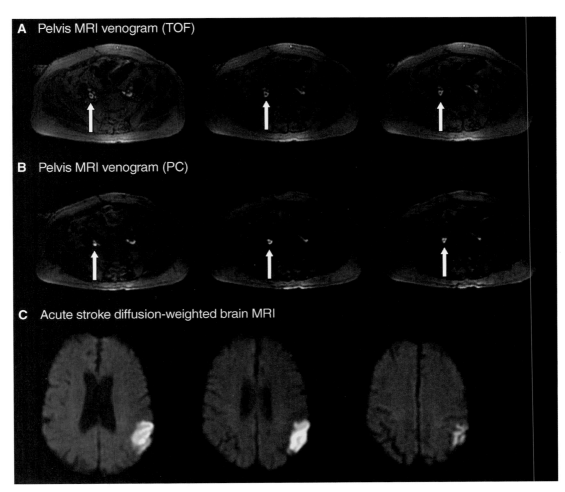

Fig. 1. A 78-year-old man with rectal adenocarcinoma presented with acute ischemic stroke. Evaluation including carotid duplex, transcranial Doppler, and transthoracic echocardiogram with agitated saline contrast injection was unremarkable except for the presence of a PFO. Leg vein duplex study was unremarkable. An MRI venogram of the pelvis was performed 3.5 days after stroke onset. (*A*) A dilated right common iliac vein with a murally based, intraluminal hypointensity of 15 mm length (*arrows*) was present on three contiguous slices from a time-of-flight venographic pulse sequence. (*B*) The hypointensity was confirmed on matched slices using a phase contrast venographic pulse sequence. (*C*) The infarct involved the left parietal cortex and had the topography of an embolic insult. PC, phase contrast; TOF, time of flight.

[38]. Mas et al [29] found a stroke recurrence rate of 1% when both PFO and atrial septal aneurysm were absent versus 3.8% when both were present. A recent large, prospective study found that the combined annual rate of death or recurrent ischemic stroke among patients with cryptogenic stroke was 7.8% [6], although a substudy found that the annual rate of death/recurrent stroke after a cryptogenic stroke was not significantly different when PFO was present (7.2%) or was not present (6.4%) [25].

PFO is a common finding in normal persons. The frequency of PFO is increased among patients with a cryptogenic stroke. Several lines of evidence suggest a role for the PFO in stroke pathophysiology for some patients, particularly those with a concomitant atrial septal aneurysm. Most studies suggest that medical therapy is associated with an important risk for recurrent events after a cryptogenic stroke. New treatments to close a PFO safely are under evaluation, although a method of identifying the patients most likely to achieve long-term benefit from this intervention remains to be established. Implementation of these and other treatments to prevent TIA, stroke, and death after a diagnosis of cryptogenic stroke may be best guided by a better understanding of the causes and consequences of cryptogenic stroke.

References

[1] Gresham GE, Duncan PW, Stason WB, et al. Post-stroke rehabilitation. Rockville (MD): US Department of Health and Human Services. Public Health Service, Agency for Health Care Policy and Research, 1995.

[2] Broderick J, Brott T, Kothari R, Miller R, et al. The Greater Cincinnati/Northern Kentucky Stroke Study: preliminary first-ever and total incidence rates of stroke among blacks. Stroke 1998;29:415–21.

[3] American Heart Association Stroke Statistics. Available at: http://www.americanheart.org/presenter.jhtml?identifier=4725.

[4] Sacco RL, Ellenberg JH, Mohr JP, et al. Infarcts of undetermined cause: the NINCDS Stroke Data Bank. Ann Neurol 1989;25:382–90.

[5] Mohr JP, Caplan LR, Melski JW, et al. The Harvard Cooperative Stroke Registry: a prospective registry of patients hospitalized with stroke. Neurology 1978;28:754–62.

[6] Mohr JP, Thompson JLP, Lazar RM, et al. A comparison of warfarin and aspirin for the prevention of recurrent ischemic stroke. N Engl J Med 2001;345:1444–51.

[7] The Publications Committee for the Trial of ORG 10172 in Acute Stroke Treatment (TOAST) Investigators. Low molecular weight heparinoid, ORG 10172 (Danaparoid), and outcome after acute ischemic stroke. JAMA 1998;279:1265–72.

[8] The National Institute of Neurological Disorders and Stroke rt-PA Stroke Study Group. Tissue plasminogen activator for acute ischemic stroke. N Engl J Med 1995;333:1581–7.

[9] Albers GW, Amarenco P, Easton JD, et al. Antithrombotic and thrombolytic therapy for ischemic stroke. Chest 2001;119:300S–20S.

[10] Cabanes L, Mas JL, Cohen A, et al. Atrial septal aneurysm and patent foramen ovale as risk factors for cryptogenic stroke in patients less than 55 years of age. A study using transesophageal echocardiography. Stroke 1993;24:1865–73.

[11] Mohr JP. Cryptogenic stroke. N Engl J Med 1988;318:1197–8.

[12] Overell JR, Bone I, Lees KR. Interatrial septal abnormalities and stroke: a meta-analysis of case-control studies. Neurology 2000;55:1172–9.

[13] Thompson T, Evans W. Paradoxical embolism. Q J Med 1930;23:135–52.

[14] Hagen PT, Scholz DG, Edwards WD. Incidence and size of patent foramen ovale during the first 10 decades of life: an autopsy study of 965 normal hearts. Mayo Clin Proc 1984;59:17–20.

[15] Lechat P, Mas JL, Lascault G. Prevalence of patent foramen ovale in patients with stroke. N Engl J Med 1988;318:1148–52.

[16] Hausmann D, Mugge A, Becht I, et al. Diagnosis of patent foramen ovale by transesophageal echocardiography and association with cerebral and peripheral embolic events. Am J Cardiol 1992;70:668–72.

[17] Jeanrenaud X, Bogousslavsky J, Payot M, et al. Patent foramen ovale and cerebral infarct in young patients. Schweiz Med Wochenschr 1990;120:823–9.

[18] Di Tullio M, Sacco RL, Gopal A, et al. Patent foramen ovale as a risk factor for cryptogenic stroke. Ann Intern Med 1992;117:461–5.

[19] Job FP, Ringelstein EB, Grafen Y, et al. Comparison of transcranial contrast Doppler sonography and transesophageal contrast echocardiography for the detection of patent foramen ovale in young stroke patients. Am J Cardiol 1994;74:381–4.

[20] Klotzsch C, Janssen G, Berlit P. Transesophageal echocardiography and contrast-TCD in the detection of a patent foramen ovale. Neurology 1994;44:1603–6.

[21] Petty GW, Khandheria BK, Chu C-P, et al. Patent foramen ovale in patients with cerebral infarction. Arch Neurol 1997;54:819–22.

[22] Homma S, Di Tullio MR, Sacco RL, et al. Characteristics of patent foramen ovale associated with cryptogenic stroke. A biplane transesophageal echocardiographic study. Stroke 1994;25:582–6.

[23] Ranoux D, Cohen A, Cabanes L, et al. Patent foramen ovale: is stroke due to paradoxical embolism? Stroke 1993;24:31–4.

[24] Steiner MM, Di Tullio MR, Rundek T, et al. Patent foramen ovale size and embolic brain imaging findings among patients with ischemic stroke. Stroke 1998;29:944–8.

[25] Homma S, Sacco RL, Di Tullio MR, et al, for the PFO in Cryptogenic Stroke Study (PICSS) Investigators. Effect of medical treatment in stroke patients with patent foramen ovale: patent foramen ovale in Cryptogenic Stroke Study. Circulation 2002;105:2625–31.

[26] Webster MW, Chancellor AM, Smith HJ, et al. Patent foramen ovale in young stroke patients. Lancet 1988:11–2.

[27] de Belder MA, Tourikis L, Leech G, et al. Risk of patent foramen ovale for thromboembolic events in all age groups. Am J Cardiol 1992;69:1316–20.

[28] De Castro S, Cartoni D, Fiorelli M, et al. Morphological and functional characteristics of patent foramen ovale and their embolic implications. Stroke 2000;31:2407–13.

[29] Mas J-L, Arquizan C, Lamy C, et al, for the Patent Foramen Ovale and Atrial Septal Aneurysm Study

Group. Recurrent cerebrovascular events associated with patent foramen ovale, atrial septal aneurysm, or both. N Engl J Med 2001;345:1740–6.

[30] Lethen H, Flachskampf FA, Schneider R, et al. Frequency of deep vein thrombosis in patients with patent foramen ovale and ischemic stroke or transient ischemic attack. Am J Cardiol 1997;80:1066–9.

[31] Ha JW, Shin MS, Kang S, et al. Enhanced detection of right-to-left shunt through patent foramen ovale by transthoracic contrast echocardiography using harmonic imaging. Am J Cardiol 2001;87:669–71, A11.

[32] Stendel R, Gramm HJ, Schroder K, et al. Transcranial Doppler ultrasonography as a screening technique for detection of a patent foramen ovale before surgery in the sitting position. Anesthesiology 2000;93:971–5.

[33] Droste DW, Lakemeier S, Wichter T, et al. Optimizing the technique of contrast transcranial Doppler ultrasound in the detection of right-to-left shunts. Stroke 2002;33:2211–6.

[34] Gin KG, Huckell VF, Pollick C. Femoral vein delivery of contrast medium enhances transthoracic echocardiographic detection of patent foramen ovale. J Am Coll Cardiol 1993;22:1994–2000.

[35] Hamann GF, Schatzer-Klotz D, Frohlig G, et al. Femoral injection of echo contrast medium may increase the sensitivity of testing for a patent foramen ovale. Neurology 1998;50:1423–8.

[36] Schuchlenz HW, Weihs W, Horner S, et al. The association between the diameter of a patent foramen ovale and the risk of embolic cerebrovascular events. Am J Med 2000;109:456–62.

[37] Kerut EK, Norfleet WT, Plotnick GD, et al. Patent foramen ovale: a review of associated conditions and the impact of physiological size. J Am Coll Cardiol 2001;38:613–23.

[38] Bogousslavsky J, Garazi S, Jeanrenaud X, et al, the Lausanne Stroke with Paradoxical Embolism Study Group. Stroke recurrence in patients with patent foramen ovale: The Lausanne Study. Neurology 1996;46:1301–5.

[39] Stollberger C, Slany J, Schuster I, et al. The prevalence of deep vein thrombosis in patients with suspected paradoxical embolism. Ann Intern Med 1993;119:461–5.

[40] Gautier JC, Durr A, Koussa S, et al. Paradoxical cerebral embolism with a patent foramen ovale. Cerebrovasc Dis 1991;1:193–202.

[41] Cramer SC, Rordorf G, Kaufman JA, et al. Clinically occult pelvic-vein thrombosis in cryptogenic stroke. Lancet 1998;351:1927–8.

[42] Cramer SC, Maki JH, Waitches GM, et al. Paradoxical emboli from calf and pelvic veins in cryptogenic stroke. J Neuroimaging 2003;13:218–23.

[43] Kelly J, Rudd A, Lewis R, et al. Venous thromboembolism after acute stroke. Stroke 2001;32:262–7.

[44] Cramer SC, Rordorf G, Maki JH, et al. Increased pelvic vein thrombi in cryptogenic stroke: results of the Paradoxical Emboli from Large Veins in Ischemic Stroke (PELVIS) study. Stroke 2004;35:46–50.

[45] Hirsh J, Hoak J. Management of deep vein thrombosis and pulmonary embolism. A statement for healthcare professionals. Council on Thrombosis (in consultation with the Council on Cardiovascular Radiology), American Heart Association. Circulation 1996;93:2212–45.

[46] Salzman EW. Venous thrombosis made easy. N Engl J Med 1986;314:847–8.

[47] Corrin B. Paradoxical embolism. Br Heart J 1964;26:549–53.

[48] Johnson BI. Paradoxical emboli. J Clin Pathol 1951;4:316–32.

[49] Spritzer CE, Arata MA, Freed KS. Isolated pelvic deep venous thrombosis: relative frequency as detected with MR imaging. Radiology 2001;219:521–5.

[50] Au VW, Walsh G, Fon G. Computed tomography pulmonary angiography with pelvic venography in the evaluation of thrombo-embolic disease. Australas Radiol 2001;45:141–5.

[51] Loud PA, Katz DS, Bruce DA, et al. Deep venous thrombosis with suspected pulmonary embolism: detection with combined CT venography and pulmonary angiography. Radiology 2001;219:498–502.

[52] Stern JB, Abehsera M, Grenet D, et al. Detection of pelvic vein thrombosis by magnetic resonance angiography in patients with acute pulmonary embolism and normal lower limb compression ultrasonography. Chest 2002;122:115–21.

[53] Greer DM, Buonanno FS. Cerebral infarction in conjunction with patent foramen ovale and May-Thurner syndrome. J Neuroimaging 2001;11:432–4.

[54] Comess KA, DeRook FA, Beach KW, et al. Transesophageal echocardiography and carotid ultrasound in patients with cerebral ischemia: prevalence of findings and recurrent stroke risk. J Am Coll Cardiol 1994;23:1598–603.

[55] Mas J-L, Zuber M, The French Study Group on Patent Foramen Ovale and Atrial Septal Aneurysm. Recurrent cerebrovascular events in patients with patent foramen ovale, atrial septal aneurysm, or both and cryptogenic stroke or transient ischemic attack. Am Heart J 1995;130:1083–8.

ELSEVIER
SAUNDERS

Cardiol Clin 23 (2005) 13–33

CARDIOLOGY
CLINICS

Percutaneous Patent Foramen Ovale Closure

John D. Carroll, MD*, Stephen Dodge, MD, Bertron M. Groves, MD

*Interventional Cardiology Section, Cardiovascular Division, University of Colorado Health Sciences Center,
4200 East Ninth Avenue, Box B-132, Denver, CO 80262, USA*

Most patients who have clinical events that are related to a patent foramen ovale (PFO) are adults. Therefore, it is expected that as this field grows, most of the procedures and investigation will involve adult interventional cardiologists. The development of devices to close PFOs percutaneously occurred in parallel with procedures to close atrial septal defects (ASDs). The pediatric interventional community has led the field of device closure of interatrial abnormalities. Individually, they first developed the skill sets that were necessary to perform the procedure. In many communities, pediatric cardiologists perform PFO and ASD closure procedures in adult patients. This article focuses on the procedure from the perspective of adult cardiology. The cognitive skills and catheter-based skills that are needed for PFO closure often are new and unique to adult cardiologists and are one focus of this article. Most attention will be focused on the two commercially available devices in the United States, the Amplatzer PFO device (AGA Medical Corp., Goldenvalley, Minnesota) and the CardioSEAL device (NMT Medical Products, Boston, Massachusetts). The two major imaging modalities of fluoroscopy and ultrasound are discussed (Figs. 1 and 2).

PFO closure is a new procedure that presents an opportunity for improved patient care and a need for caution because of many unresolved issues in the care of these patients. The challenges of beginning a program of PFO closure are outlined in Box 1.

This article also concentrates on the PFO closure that is performed by a team. During the learning curve, this team may include pediatric and adult interventional cardiologists, nurse practitioners, the cardiac catheterization laboratory staff, and often, additional professionals who are skilled in echocardiography and anesthesia. This clearly is a change from the standard coronary interventions that typically do not involve professionals from outside of the cardiac catheterization laboratory. The PFO closure procedure joins the list of rapidly developing new therapeutic procedures that involve a new device and the need to form new and diverse teams of professionals who provide new skill sets and experience.

The team composition and the performance of the procedure vary from one institution to another and within each institution over time with greater experience. On one extreme is the performance of PFO closure using general anesthesia and transesophageal guidance. At the other extreme is the use of fluoroscopy only for device placement and angiography for documentation of closure. The best approach for each institution requires assessment of local resources, experience, and the device that is being used.

PFO closure also is unique to the adult interventional cardiologist in that the benefit of the procedure is to prevent a possible recurrent noncardiac event—typically cerebral ischemia—versus the immediate relief or reduction of cardiovascular symptoms. A good contrast is direct coronary intervention in acute myocardial infarction where the value of the procedure to the patient is recognized immediately. In PFO closure, the therapeutic benefit requires longitudinal observation as is done with other kinds of risk reduction therapy. The procedure does not make the patient feel better or able to do activities that

---

* Corresponding author.
E-mail address: john.carroll@uchsc.edu
(J.D. Carroll).

0733-8651/05/$ - see front matter © 2005 Elsevier Inc. All rights reserved.
doi:10.1016/j.ccl.2004.10.010

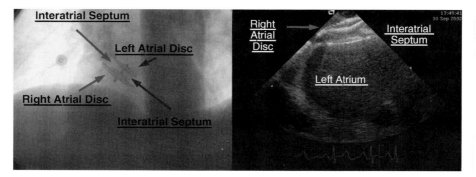

Fig. 1. (*Left*) The Amplazter PFO device is shown with its typical radiographic appearance of two discs, the smaller is in the left atrium. (*Right*) Amplatzer PFO device is shown using ultrasound, specifically intracardiac ultrasound. The interatrial septum is well-visualized by ultrasound.

have been restricted. Notable exceptions to this generalization include scuba divers who have PFOs and rare patients who have platypnea orthodeoxia (ie, hypoxemia from right-to-left shunting through a PFO without concomitant severe pulmonary hypertension).

Device closure of patent foramen ovale: overview of the device design and anatomy

A variety of PFO closure devices has been developed and tested. In the United States, two devices are commercially available. The Amplatzer PFO device is used as a representative device to discuss the design specifications that are needed for percutaneous closure of the standard PFO.

The mechanisms by which devices close a PFO are two-fold. First the device acts like a paper clip or cufflink in holding the flap of tissue—represented in embryologic development as the septum primum—against the rest of the interatrial septum. The second principle is the barrier that is provided by the two discs that are jointed together by a connecting pin. For the 25-mm Amplatzer PFO occluder, the right atrial disc is 25 mm in diameter and the left atrial disc is 18 mm (see Fig. 1, left panel). Within each disc is sewn a polyester patch that serves to occlude blood flow. Both discs have inward tension as part of the shape memory of the nitinol wire mesh which produces a compressive force between the two discs.

The anatomy of the PFO and surrounding structures is not a simple wall with a flap of tissue. Rather, there are three-dimensional distortions that require the device to have a fair degree of

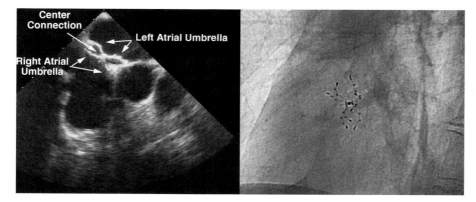

Fig. 2. (*Left panel*) Transesophageal ultrasound image. (*Right panel*) Fluoroscopic image in lateral projection. The CardioSEAL's appearance is distinctive with its stainless steel arms and cloth umbrellas. Both are successful in holding the two flaps of tissue together (ie, the septum primum and secundum) and provide additional barriers against paradoxical embolism.

Box 1. Challenges in starting a patent
foramen ovale program and performing
device closure of patent foramen ovale

Incompleteness of scientific studies
Special regulatory oversight
Uncertainties in patient selection
Learning curve challenges in procedure
    performance
High start-up costs and uncertain
    reimbursement

conformability. This is most apparent at the base of the aorta which requires the two discs to mold themselves around the aorta. On the inferoposterior aspect of the PFO the septum may be thin and hypermobile which requires the two discs to clamp down on the thin structure. Extensive overlap of the flap and minimal excursion, as with a tunnel anatomy, can be unsuitable for the short center pin that connects the two discs. PFO devices, therefore, must be versatile and flexible given the diversity of patient size, PFO size, and variations of shape of the septum and surrounding structures.

Device closure of patent foramen ovale: published reports

There are numerous single and multi-center reports of experience in PFO closure using a variety of percutaneously implanted devices. The following discussion highlights some of the key reports that provide a comprehensive state of the field in early 2004.

Six centers in Germany, one center in Switzerland, and two centers in the United States have published the largest case series that reported immediate and long-term results of percutaneous PFO closure. Sievert et al [1] at the Cardiovascular Center Bethanien, Frankfurt, Germany reported the largest single series of patients who underwent percutaneous PFO closure. Percutaneous PFO closure was performed in 281 consecutive patients who had a history of cryptogenic stroke, transient ischemic attack (TIA), or other peripheral embolic event. Seven different devices were used (35% PFO-Star, 20% Amplatzer, 13% CardioSEAL & StarFLEX, 12% Helex [W.L. Gore and Associates, Flaggstaff, New Mexico], 9% Sideris buttoned device Sideris [Custom Medical Devices, Amarillo, Texas], 7% Angel wings

[Microvena Corp., White Bear Lake, Minnesota], and 4% anal septal defect occlusion system [ASDOS], [Osypka Corp., Germany]). The procedural success rate was 100%. Procedural complications occurred in 3%, including one death from septicemia, device embolization (<1%), and atrial fibrillation. Residual interatrial shunting was present by transesophageal echocardiography (TEE) in 5.5% after 6 months. The actuarial risk of a recurrent clinical embolic event was 4.3% at 1 year and 5.9% at 3 years.

Braun et al [2] reported the outcomes of percutaneous PFO closure from four centers in Germany in 276 consecutive patients who had a history of cryptogenic stroke or TIA and PFO [2]. The PFO-Star device was used in all patients. Procedural success rate was 100%. Procedural complications occurred in 4%, including device embolization (<1%), TIA, atrial fibrillation, reversible atrio-ventricular (AV) block, and reversible ST-segment elevation due to presumed air emboli. Residual shunt was present by TEE in 17% after 1 month, 4% after 6 months, and 1% after 1 and 2 years. The actuarial risk of a recurrent clinical embolic event was 1.7% at 1 year.

Bruch et al [3] at Unfallkrankenhaus, Berlin, Germany reported the results of percutaneous PFO and ASD closure in 66 consecutive patients who had a history of cryptogenic stroke, TIA, or other peripheral embolic event. PFO was present in 82% of patients and ASD was present in 18% of patients. Five different devices were used (61% Amplatzer PFO, 33% Amplatzer ASD, 3% PFO-Star, 1.5% CardioSEAL, and 1.5% StarFLEX). The procedural success rate was 100%. There were no procedural complications. Three patients (5%) developed fever postprocedure without sequelae. Two patients (3%) developed atrial fibrillation postprocedure. Residual shunt was present by TEE in 3% after 3 months and in none after 6 and 12 months. There were no recurrent clinical embolic events over 112.2 patient-years of follow-up (range, 5 weeks to 43 months).

Wahl et al [4] from the Swiss Cardiovascular Center, Bern, Switzerland reported the results of percutaneous PFO closure in 152 consecutive patients who had a history of cryptogenic stroke, TIA, or other peripheral embolic event. Six different devices were used (30% Amplatzer PFO, 29% PFO-Star, 20% Sideris buttoned device, 7% CardioSEAL & StarFLEX, 7% Amplatzer ASD, and 7% Angel wings). Procedural success rate was 99%. Procedural complications occurred in 7% of patients, including device embolization (2.6%), cardiac tamponade in one patient, air embolism, and femoral AV fistula. Residual shunt was present in 21% by TEE after 6 months. Of those, 41% had the Sideris buttoned device and 34% had the PFO-Star device. The actuarial risk of a recurrent clinical embolic event was 4.9% at 1 year and 9.4% at 2 and 6 years. Residual shunt was a risk factor for recurrent embolism (Relative Risk, 5.3; 95% confidence interval, 1.3–21.0; $P = .02$). The actuarial risk of a recurrent clinical embolic event for patients who did not have residual shunt was 1.9% at 1 year and 5.8% at 2 and 6 years.

Martin et al [5] at the Massachusetts General Hospital reported the results of percutaneous PFO closure in 110 consecutive patients who had a history of cryptogenic stroke, TIA, or other peripheral embolic event. Two different devices were used (70% Sideris buttoned device, 30% CardioSEAL). Procedural success rate was 100%. Procedural complications occurred in 6% of patients, including device embolization in one patient, cardiac tamponade in one patient, atrial fibrillation, and supraventricular tachycardia. Residual shunt was present in 56% of patients immediately postprocedure. Residual shunt was present by transthoracic echocardiography (TTE) in 47% after 6 months and 33% after 12 months. The actuarial risk of a recurrent clinical embolic event was 2.1% at 5 years. Recurrent embolism was not related to the presence of a residual shunt.

Du et al [6] at the University of Chicago Children's Hospital reported the results of percutaneous PFO closure in 18 consecutive patients who had a history of cryptogenic stroke or TIA. Three different devices were used (39% Angel wings, 33% Amplatzer ASD, and 28% Amplatzer PFO). Procedural success rate was 100%. There were no procedural complications. Residual shunt was present in 33% of patients immediately postprocedure. Residual shunt was present by TTE or TEE in none of the patients after 6 and 12 months. There were no recurrent clinical embolic events over 2.2 ± 1.8 years of follow-up.

The earlier multi-center experience with the ASDOS device at seven centers in Germany and Switzerland was reported by Sievert et al [7] and included 46 patients who had a history of cryptogenic stroke or TIA and PFO. For the entire cohort of 200 patients who had ASD or PFO, the procedural success rate was 87%. Procedural complications occurred in 4% of patients, including device embolization (1%), device entrapment (<1%), cardiac tamponade (1%), air embolism

(1%), and femoral hematoma that required surgery (1%). Late atrial wall perforation occurred in 1.5% of patients. Infectious endocarditis developed in 1% of patients. Residual shunt was present in 37% of patients immediately postprocedure. Residual shunt was present by TTE or TEE in 28% of patients after 12 months. The recurrent clinical embolic event rate for patients who had PFO was 2.2% over a follow-up of 49 patient-years.

The case series that were outlined above suggest an annual stroke or TIA recurrence rate of approximately 2% to 3% following percutaneous PFO closure. No randomized studies of percutaneous PFO closure versus medical therapy for secondary prevention of paradoxical thromboembolization has been completed. Cohort studies suggested an annual stroke or TIA recurrence rate of approximately 4% to 6% with medical therapy (ie, antiplatelet agents or oral anticoagulation) [8–11]. Case series of surgical PFO closure reported an annual stroke or TIA recurrence rate that ranges from 0% to nearly 20% [8,12–14]. The largest series of 91 patients who underwent surgical PFO closure at the Mayo Clinic reported an annual stroke or TIA recurrence rate of 7.5% [12].

Several points need to be made when evaluating these studies. The devices that were used include several that did not perform well in terms of yielding a complete closure, device embolization, and other major complications. Major complications are now rare with currently used devices and complete closure is in the 95% range when performed by experienced teams. Complete closure only can be judged by the more sensitive TEE approach that involves the Valsalva maneuver and, optimally, microbubble solution entering from the inferior vena cava (IVC), as opposed to arm-based injections. Finally, recurrent neurologic events need to be understood more completely. In some patients they may represent an incorrect diagnosis of the initial neurologic events being due to a paradoxical embolism. In other patients, they may represent device thrombosis and clot embolization or incomplete closure with paradoxical embolization.

Current randomized trials to assess device closure

There are at least four active or planned randomized clinical trials to compare device closure with medical therapy at the time of this article's preparation. Two are evaluating the

Amplatzer PFO Occluder and one planned trial will evaluate the StarFLEX device, a newer generation device that was derived from the Cardio-SEAL device. A third trial in the United States is using the Cardia device (Cardia Inc., Burnsville, Minnesota).

The Patent Foramen Ovale in Cryptogenic Embolism Trial is the only trial that has been enrolling patients since early 2000; however, it has had slower than expected enrollment. It is a multicenter, multi-national randomized clinical trial that compares the efficacy of percutaneous PFO closure using the Amplatzer PFO Occluder with best medical treatment in patients who have PFO and paradoxical embolism. Patients who are randomized to device closure are treated with aspirin plus clopidogrel for 3 to 6 months after device implantation. Patients who are randomized into the best medical treatment arm of the study do not undergo percutaneous device closure of the PFO, but are treated with antithrombotic medication. Because there is no consensus on the most effective medical therapy in preventing recurrent stroke or TIA in patients who have PFO and paradoxical embolism, the choice of antithrombotic therapy—oral anticoagulation or antiplatelet therapy, as judged to be the best medical treatment—will be decided by the treating physician. The primary objective of this study is to investigate whether percutaneous PFO closure (using the Amplatzer PFO Occluder) is equal or superior to best medical treatment in the prevention of symptomatic, recurrent thromboembolism. The combined primary end point consists of death, stroke, TIA, and peripheral embolism. Patients who experience a primary end point event during the study period do not have to continue the treatment that was allocated at the time of randomization. Cross over from medical treatment to PFO device closure or from PFO device closure to additional antithrombotic treatment will be allowed in case of a primary end point event. All patients will continue to be followed for further events after an initial primary end point, according to the study protocol, for the total duration of this study. The secondary end points include new arrhythmia, myocardial infarction, rehospitalization related to PFO or its treatment, device problems (eg, dislodgment, structural failure, infection, thrombosis), and bleeding complications that are due to antithrombotic therapy. Further outcome measures are a quality of life assessment and employment status. The data collected also should allow an estimate of cost and cost benefit of the treatments.

The RESPECT Trial (Randomized Evaluation of Recurrent Stroke Comparing PFO Closure to Established Current Standard of Care Treatment) is a United States trial of the Amplatzer PFO device. The RESPECT Trial will investigate whether percutaneous PFO closure is better than or equivalent to current standard-of-care medical therapy in the prevention of recurrent symptomatic stroke. The preliminary design is a multi-center, randomized, active control, blinded adjudicated outcome, clinical trial with a statistical analysis of noninferiority. The sample size is planned to be 420 patients (210 per study arm). Patients will be 18 to 55 years old who have PFO and have had a cryptogenic stroke within the last 3 months. Patients will be assigned randomly to best medical therapy or PFO closure with the Amplatzer PFO Occluder. The primary end point is recurrent symptomatic cryptogenic stroke or cardiovascular death. The secondary efficacy end point is complete closure of the interatrial defect at the 6-month follow-up based upon TEE assessment of residual shunting. The primary safety end point is all adverse events.

Although randomized clinical trials are needed, there are several challenges for trial design. The first is the medication that is used in the control arm. Warfarin is used widely for presumed paradoxical embolism; however, recent medical trials in stroke secondary prevention failed to show its superiority over aspirin. These trials did not randomize prospectively patients who had cryptogenic stroke that was presumed to be secondary to PFO. The next trial design challenge is whether the device should show superiority to medical therapy or equivalency or noninferiority. Finally, the measured events during treatment may be stroke or stroke and TIAs.

Current indications for device closure of patent foramen ovale

Selection of patients who would benefit without an unreasonable risk constitutes the framework for discussing current indications for PFO closure. Translating this simple statement into individual patient selection is not simple. The four key elements in this decision process include the clinical event, the exclusion of other possible etiologies that might cause or contribute to the event, the anatomic and physiologic characterization of the PFO, and whether events have occurred despite medical therapy. These topics are discussed elsewhere in this issue.

The number of patients who may need PFO closure is difficult to determine because of the early stages of clinical experience and the lack of randomized clinical trial guidance. A conservative estimate would predict that several thousand patients per year in the Unites States present with a PFO and recurrent embolic events, despite adequate anticoagulation. The highest estimate might predict that 30,000 to 100,000 patients per year have a cryptogenic stroke that is associated with a PFO. At the extreme would be the 20% to 30% of the population who has a PFO, although closure of a PFO in an asymptomatic individual is not supported by current data [15–18]. Investigations have started to study the possible role of PFO closure in the treatment of migraine headaches, a malady affecting millions. A summary of current indications for PFO closure is provided in Box 2.

Informed consent and patient and family education

Closure of PFO requires an informed consent from the patient who understands the following issues: the nature of the person's illness; the nature of the proposed treatment, including the likelihood of attaining success as well as failure; possible complications; and alternative treatments available to the patient. For PFO closure there are two special considerations in obtaining informed consent. The first relates to the mental state of the patient and the second is the challenge of informing patients and family in an area of medical uncertainty.

The patient who has a PFO that is referred for closure recently had one or more cerebrovascular events. Most patients have recovered completely and are mentally competent to give informed consent; however, some patients may have residual abnormalities that involve cognition, especially when seen within days to weeks of a neurologic event. It is the responsibility of the neurologist and interventional cardiologist to ascertain the ability of the patient to provide informed consent. The patient may have family members and friends who can provide insight regarding the patient's mental status and participate in the informed consent process.

Also, most of these patients recently have had their first encounter with a serious personal medical problem. Most are coming to grips with the reality that they have a heart abnormality in addition to a stroke. The frequent young to

---

Box 2. Indications for percutaneous patent foramen ovale closure

United States Food and Drug Administration approved indications for patent foramen ovale closure under humanitarian device exemption regulations
The CardioSEAL Occluder and Amplatzer PFO Occluder are indicted for the following:
Closure of PFO in patients who have recurrent cryptogenic stroke due to presumed paradoxical embolism through a PFO and who have failed conventional drug therapy.

Other patent foramen ovale closure "off-label" uses or indications that are under investigation
Cryptogenic stroke due to presumed paradoxical embolism through a PFO
   After the first clinical event
   Patients who have contraindications to anticoagulant treatment
   As an alternative to medical therapy or surgical closure
Cryptogenic TIA due to presumed paradoxical embolism through a PFO
Presumed paradoxical peripheral or coronary arterial embolism through a PFO
Cryptogenic stroke, TIA, or peripheral or coronary embolism due to presumed paradoxical embolism through a PFO that is associated with a hypercoagulability state
Divers who have a PFO who are at risk of clinical events that are related to paradoxical embolism through a PFO during decompression [19]
Systemic deoxygenation due to right-to-left shunting through a PFO in the absence of severe pulmonary hypertension (eg, platypnea orthodeoxia, right ventricular infarction) [20]
Migraine headaches accompanied by aura
Posttraumatic fat embolism syndrome with cerebral embolism by way of PFO

middle-aged nature of this patient group and the suddenness of their transition into being a patient impact upon their expectations and hopes. Many are searching for a "quick-fix" and may be inclined to view a device implantation as an avenue to disease cure and, alternatively, perceive life-long medication as a huge barrier to their lifestyle. It is the physician's responsibility to present the data on treatment options in an unbiased fashion.

Added to this psychologic state is the medical reality that PFO closure is a new procedure with many unresolved issues. The lack of randomized trial data requires the informing physician to explain carefully the role of percutaneous closure versus other therapies. The narrow indication for PFO closure under the Humanitarian Device Exemption regulations must be understood to explain to the patient that (1) the devices that have been approved are no longer investigational; (2) the approval primarily demonstrates the relative safety of the device and the procedure; (3) nonrandomized, single center studies showed effectiveness against historic controls; and (4) broader, randomized studies of effectiveness are pending. The few alternatives for the patient who has recurrent events—despite optimal medical management—must also be stated clearly. Surgical closure remains an option although it is chosen rarely.

Device closure has the goal of prevention of further arterial embolic events, not correction of neurologic deficits that have occurred as a result of earlier embolic events. This must be stated firmly during the process of informed consent. The frequency of failure of the device to close the defect also must be stated. Some published studies [4,6] showed an association between recurrent neurologic events and residual shunts.

The listing of potential complications during the process of informed consent does not have to be as comprehensive as has been reported in the literature. The potential complications must be explained in adequate detail to allow the patient to understand the likelihood and nature of minor and major complications. These fall into several categories as outlined in Box 3.

Most patients and their families are eager to learn more about the cause of their neurologic event, details of device closure, and long-term prognosis. Educational materials are meager. Web-based resources are available and handouts can be obtained from the device manufacturers (www.amplatzer.com and www.nmtmedical.com). A patient education document is available from the University of Colorado Health Sciences Center at www.uhcolorado/cardiaccath.edu.

Operator skills and equipment needed

Box 4 lists the operator skills and cardiac catheterization laboratory equipment that are needed for PFO closure. Note that some skills are not routine for the adult interventional cardiologist and cardiac catheterization laboratory staff.

Box 3. Complications from percutaneous patent foramen ovale device closure

Bleeding related to vascular access—because most procedures involve only venous access, bleeding is uncommon and generally minor.
Complications that are associated with intracardiac implantation of the devices:
    Premature atrial contractions are not common but may be frightening to the patient.
    Sustained supraventricular or atrial fibrillation is uncommon.
    Arterial air embolism with cardiac or neurologic manifestations, including ST-segment elevation and myocardial ischemia
    Cardiac or systemic venous vascular perforation
    Device embolization
Major complications, including stroke, myocardial infarction, death
Complications related to general anesthesia, TEE, angiography, and intracardiac echocardiography (ICE), if performed
Complications during follow-up
    Arrhythmia in the first 6 weeks after the procedure with a 4% to 5% incidence of premature atrial contractions and 1% atrial fibrillation that usually IS transient
    Device thrombosis
    Device degeneration that is device-specific

Box 4. General and procedure-specific skills and equipment that are needed for patent foramen ovale closure

Conscious sedation and general anesthesia skills and equipment
Knowledge and clinical skills for pre-, intra-, and postprocedure antithrombotic and
    antiplatelet strategies including:
    Diagnosis and treatment of hypercoagulable states
    Intraprocedure anticoagulation and monitoring
    Bridging off and on warfarin with periprocedural heparins
    Device thrombosis prophylaxis, recognition, and management skills
Advanced right heart catheterization skills and equipment
    Venous access/exit skills and insertion of multiple large devices
    Performance of hemodynamic studies
    Performance of intracardiac and pulmonary AV shunt evaluation
    Familiarity with IVC filters
Transseptal catheterization skills and equipment
    Catheter crossing of PFO and manipulation into pulmonary veins
    Performance of needle puncture of interatrial septum and catheter insertion into the left
        atrium
    Prevention of air embolism and its recognition and treatment
    Prevention of pulmonary venous perforation and irritation that causes coughing and
        generation of negative intrathoracic pressures.
Radiography-based skills in fluoroscopy and angiography with high-resolution digital
    imaging and storage
    Right and left atrial angiography
    Determination of optimal views for PFO closure and related structures
Ultrasound skills and equipment—TEE or ICE
    Manipulation of transducer/probe/catheter
    Optimization of images and Doppler data
    Interpretation of images and Doppler data
    Performance of agitated saline studies
Device-related skills, device inventory, and delivery catheters
    In-depth understanding and experience of PFO device sizing, preparation, use, and
        troubleshooting
    In-depth understanding of relevant anatomy and experience in device positioning in
        anatomic variants
    Availability and skills in implantation of ASD closure devices
Device retrieval and removal skills and equipment
Pericardiocentesis skills and equipment
    Recognition and management of hemopericardium

General arrhythmia monitoring, management skills, and equipment
Sterile technique, knowledge of antibiotic prophylaxis, and management skills of access site
    and device infections
Recognition and management skills for intraprocedural and postprocedural changes in
    mental status or appearance of a neurologic deficit

Patient preparation

Patient preparation is generally the same as used for cardiac catheterization procedures. In addition, the initiation of aspirin 2 to 3 days preprocedure is routine in most patients. Most patients have been taking warfarin; typically, this should be discontinued 3 to 4 days preprocedure to allow an international normalized ratio to decrease to less than 1.6. Patient-specific circumstances may warrant the preprocedural usage of heparin or low molecular weight heparins.

Cardiac catheterization laboratory set-up

Two major issues are involved in the set-up of the cardiac catheterization laboratory for PFO closure. The first relates to the need for ultrasound guidance. The second relates to the equipment and its preparation.

PFO closure is performed using a combination of fluoroscopy, angiography, and ultrasound. Although some experienced centers have discontinued the use of any ultrasound for routine PFO closure, they are the exception not the rule; other experienced centers believe that ultrasound is indispensable. The addition of ultrasound technology and skills to the cardiac catheterization laboratory environment is different from the traditional intravascular ultrasound for coronary interventions. Ultrasound guidance for PFO closure

can be provided by TEE or ICE. The acquisition and subsequent presentation of these images to the operator must be convenient to allow the nearly simultaneous review of live fluoroscopy and ultrasound images (Fig. 3). A mounted, dedicated monitor on the tableside monitor bank is optional for this procedure.

If TEE is used, there must be patient access for the physician who is performing the TEE. Furthermore, TEE during the procedure exposes the patient to airway compromise because of the supine position. Usually, the TEE probe is in place long enough to produce discomfort for the patient. Therefore, most institutions that use TEE guidance use general anesthesia that is induced by an anesthesiology team. This addition of extra people and equipment substantially alters the environment of the cardiac catheterization laboratory. Planning and execution of this team approach presents unique challenges. Altering the radiograph gantry positioning amid the additional personnel and equipment presents an additional challenge.

The recent availability of echocardiographic imaging that is provided by intracardiac ultrasound has resulted in a major improvement in patient comfort, recovery time, and efficiency of procedure performance. The advantages of the ICE-based approach to PFO closure include (1) the use of only conscious sedation and local anesthesia, which decreases patient discomfort

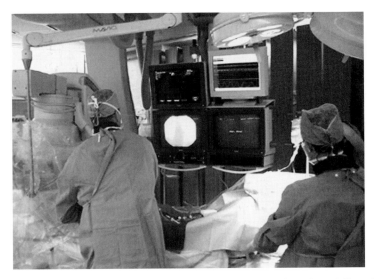

Fig. 3. A monitor for ICE images (*upper left*) is next to the live fluoroscopy monitor (*lower left*) to allow optimal use of simultaneous modalities to guide PFO closure. The physiologic monitor (*upper right*) and roadmap monitor (*lower right*) complete the tableside presentation of key data.

and morbidity; (2) the ability of the interventional cardiologist to perform the ultrasound imaging, and (3) the excellent quality of images during device deployment. The disadvantages include the cost of the ICE catheter and the ultrasound unit and the new skills that are needed for image acquisition and interpretation by the interventional cardiologist and his/her cardiac catheterization staff who serve as surrogates for experienced TEE sonographers. After these skills are acquired, the entire procedure becomes simpler to schedule and perform and is less expensive.

Procedure performance

The general steps that are involved in a PFO closure procedure are outlined in Box 5. The following discussion concentrates on relevant details of each of these steps. Procedure performance at the University of Colorado Hospital, as outlined here, constantly undergoes improvements and modifications. Therefore, this serves as a guideline for procedure performance that needs to be updated, customized for different institutions, and individualized for the diversity of patients who are encountered in practice. For device-specific tasks, the reader is referred to the manufacturers' instructions for use.

Sedation, anesthesia, and venous access

Intravenous versed and fentanyl are titrated to provide conscious sedation and analgesia.

Box 5. Steps in performance of a patent foramen ovale closure procedure

Sedation, anesthesia, and venous access
Anticoagulation, infection prophylaxis, and patient monitoring
Initial diagnostic studies
Catheter-crossing of PFO
Sizing of PFO and selection of device size
Device preparation
Delivery catheter placement and positioning
Device insertion and deployment
Device release and assessment of device placement
Final measurements and exit of venous access

Standard local anesthesia is achieved with lidocaine infiltration of the right groin region over the femoral vein. Two sheaths are inserted in the right femoral vein after gaining access by way of separate needle sticks. An 11 French (Fr) short sheath is used for the ICE catheter and an 8 to 9 Fr sheath is used for the initial right heart catheterization and the subsequent PFO device delivery catheter. The most convenient access site is the right femoral vein; the left femoral vein is an acceptable alternative. Unlike the positioning of devices for large ASDs, the delivery catheter for PFO device placement does not have to be precisely perpendicular to the plane of the interatrial septum.

Anticoagulation, infection prophylaxis, and patient monitoring

Anticoagulation during the PFO closure procedure is important. The goal is an activated clotting time (ACT) of approximately 250 seconds, although no study has been done to determine the optimal level of anticoagulation. The chief concerns are thrombus formation on intracardiac guidewires, catheters, and devices during the implantation. A common initial dose of intravenous unfractionated heparin is 60 units per kilogram of body weight. The timing of this heparin bolus may be delayed if a transseptal needle puncture is needed to gain entry into the left atrium when the PFO is associated with a slitlike tunnel.

Implantation of a permanent cardiac device raises the issue of peri-procedural antibiotic administration. Although the procedure is performed as sterilely as possible, the minimal risk of giving one to two doses of an intravenous antibiotic has resulted in the usage of a cephalosporin or vancomycin during device implantation in many institutions.

From venous access through venous exit, continuous patient monitoring in the cardiac catheterization laboratory is essential. At a minimum, the technologic component should consist of multiple electrocardiographic leads, noninvasive systemic arterial pressure monitoring, noninvasive oxygen saturation monitoring, and neurologic mental status observation.

Initial diagnostic studies

A baseline right heart catheterization with measurement of pressure to exclude unexpected pulmonary hypertension is a reasonable diagnostic study to perform before all PFO closures. The measurement of right- and left-sided filling pressure, including a pulmonary capillary wedge pressure or direct left atrial pressure measurement, is necessary to determine the patient's volume status. Dehydration with low filling pressures that become negative during inspiration represents a major risk factor for air embolism that is treated easily with intravenous volume expansion before the insertion of large delivery sheaths into the left atrium. Occasionally, it is appropriate to quantify baseline left-to-right shunting through a large PFO by collecting an oximetry series. The measurement of pulmonary venous saturation is necessary to evaluate patients who are referred for PFO closure because of right-to-left shunting that results in systemic oxygen desaturation.

The routine performance of preclosure injection of agitated saline/blood for detection of right-to-left shunting through the PFO is not necessary because most patients should have had this done during an initial precatheterization transesophageal ultrasound. In some patients, there may be a need to perform an additional bubble study because the injection of agitated saline from the femoral vein or is superior in diagnostic sensitivity to upper body venous injection. Blood flow from the is directed at the interatrial septum, especially in the presence of a prominent eustachian valve. In addition, agitated saline injection can be performed easily into the pulmonary artery to assess for a shunt through a pulmonary AV fistula.

Angiography usually is not necessary during PFO closure. Adult interventional cardiologists may not be familiar with angiography of a PFO and ASDs. The indication for this may be a preclosure clarification of interatrial anatomy and the presence of right-to-left shunting. Postprocedure, some operators use angiography to clarify device position and closure before release of the delivery cable. The use of fluoroscopy and angiography as an alternative to TEE or ICE is being evaluated in several centers. To clarify the right side of the interatrial septum, a hand injection of contrast into a large bore catheter in the lower right atrium may be adequate. A power injection is needed for a more robust opacification, including adequate image quality during the levo phase (ie, after contrast has completed the transpulmonary vascular transit). The best gantry position to observe the right and left atrial borders along the interatrial septum is left anterior oblique

(LAO)–cranial angulation, approximately LAO 30° and cranial 30°.

The ultrasound visualization of the interatrial septum with a TEE probe or an ICE catheter completes the diagnostic phase of the procedure. Imaging should verify the location and the nature of the PFO and the presence or absence of an atrial septal aneurysm and exclude the coexistence of an ASD. The ICE catheter tip is placed in the lateral aspect of the right atrium, manipulated to provide an optimal image of the PFO, and "parked" to guide the subsequent steps of PFO closure.

Catheter-crossing of patent foramen ovale

A PFO is crossed easily in approximately 95% of patients who undergo a closure procedure (Fig. 4). Approaching the PFO from the with a standard "J" tipped 0.035" to 0.038" guidewire inside a multi-purpose catheter results in immediate crossing with minimal operator manipulation. In some patients, the catheter must be directed posteromedially to allow the guidewire to cross the PFO. The tip of the guidewire usually enters the left upper pulmonary vein (desired) or the left atrial appendage (not desired). Entry into the left atrial appendage typically is recognized by: (1) tactile resistance to further advancement with tip curling, (2) the tip of the guidewire never continuing beyond the fluoroscopic border of the heart, and (3) the production of premature atrial contractions. To direct the guidewire tip into the left upper pulmonary vein may require using the multi-purpose catheter to cross the PFO while the guidewire is retracted inside the catheter. The catheter is torqued superiorly to redirect the guidewire tip away from the left atrial appendage. Occasionally, the guidewire tip will enter a left lower pulmonary vein. Advancement of the tip of the guidewire or any catheter excessively deep into the pulmonary venous system with accompanying resistance should be avoided. Deep penetration of a pulmonary vein may provoke coughing which can cause the generation of negative intrathoracic pressures with the accompanying risk of air entry into a catheter or delivery sheath. In addition, perforation of a pulmonary vein is a potential complication.

A small subset of PFOs may be more challenging to cross. The first group consists of patients who have a distorted anatomy with an abnormal plane of the interatrial septum. A Judkin's right coronary catheter tip shape may be useful in some of these patients. A second group consists of patients who have tunnel PFOs. Once again, a catheter with a more angulated tip may help. A hydrophilic guidewire also may allow easier crossing of these anatomic variants of PFO position and type. TEE or ICE imaging provides useful visual guidance in crossing some PFOs. The radiopaque "J" tipped guidewire is seen easily on ultrasound images (see Fig. 4).

Making a transseptal needle puncture is an option for PFO closure when the PFO is not crossed readily. Thus, transseptal needle puncture equipment and technical skills should be available to the interventional cardiologist who develops a PFO closure program. Parenthetically, the operator should consider difficulty in crossing the PFO as a possible indication that the defect may not be present. False positive bubble studies and technically inadequate TEE studies may result in a patient being referred for a planned closure procedure where no PFO is found and the procedure is aborted.

The transeptal approach can be performed under ICE guidance with subsequent placement of the PFO closure device. As shown in Fig. 5, the puncture site must be close enough to the PFO such that the deployed device overlaps the PFO. The transseptal approach is used by some operators when a tunnel PFO is encountered or more broadly applied because of the tight fit of the device arms against the septum.

Sizing of patent foramen ovale and selection of device size

The use of a sizing balloon during the PFO closure procedure is common, although of uncertain value in the opinion of some experts. Balloon sizing is performed by slowly and gently inflating a manufacturer's sizing balloon in the PFO using an extra stiff guidewire across the PFO with its distal end in a left pulmonary vein. The waist that appears with balloon inflation can be

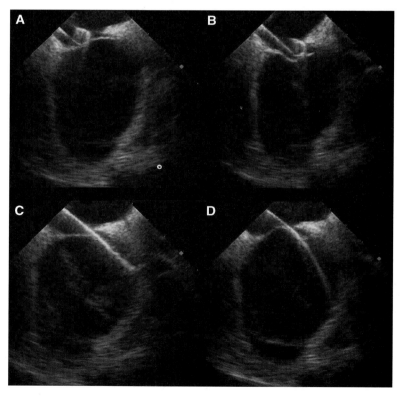

Fig. 4. These ICE images show four time points in the crossing of a PFO with a "J" tipped 0.038" guidewire. As the tip approaches the PFO from the IVC (*A*) the septum primum is deformed and opens the PFO (*B*). Further advancement results in the crossing of the PFO into the left atrium (*C*) with the final location of the guidewire tip in the left upper pulmonary vein (*D, lower right*).

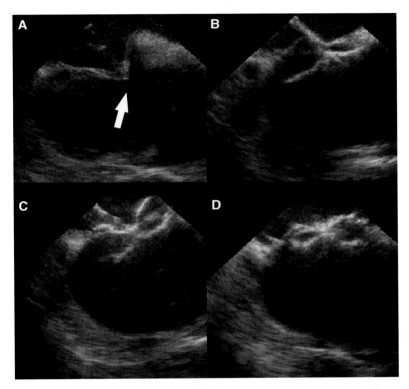

Fig. 5. An alternative approach to PFO closure involves the performance of a transeptal puncture for device deployment, rather than deploying the device in the PFO itself. Under ICE guidance, a transseptal puncture is performed in a location close to the PFO. (*A*) Note the tenting of the septum (*arrow*). Subsequently, the device is deployed, left side first (*B*), then the right atrial side (*C*), with delivery cable release (*D*).

measured by ultrasound or digital fluoroscopic images with appropriate calibration. The device size is chosen, using the manufacturer's recommendations, based on the measured diameter of the opened PFO. Finally, the waist may be discrete, which indicates a simple PFO, or more lengthy, which suggests a tunnel-like PFO. The finding of a tunnel PFO leads some operators to perform a transseptal needle puncture to place a more centrally located perpendicular device that overlaps the PFO, rather than using the PFO itself for the location of the center connection of the device which may be tilted by the tunnel. Other measurements of the patient's atrial anatomy can be made to estimate where the edge of the device will reach.

The additional presence of an atrial septal aneurysm frequently prompts the selection of a larger closure device. This practice, although used widely, has not been documented to improve the rate of PFO closure or the reduction in

subsequent clinical events. It is hoped that the usefulness of encapsulation of the atrial septal aneurysm by a larger device will be studied in future clinical trials.

The current selection of CardioSEAL Occluder devices includes diameters that are 17 mm, 28 mm, 33 mm, and 44 mm. A 28 mm device is used most commonly; however, a 33 mm device is used frequently for a PFO with an atrial septal aneurysm. The size refers to the dimension of the square umbrella on the right and left atrial sides.

The current selection of Amplatzer PFO Occluder devices includes diameters that are 18 mm, 25 mm, and 35 mm; the 25 mm size is used most commonly. The size refers to the diameter of the right atrial disc; the left atrial disk is smaller.

Device preparation

The CardioSEAL Occluder device (Fig. 6) and the Amplatzer PFO Occluder device (Fig. 7) are

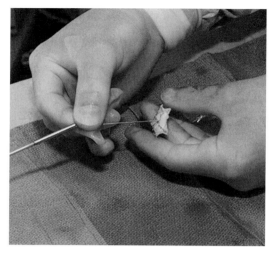

Fig. 6. Attachment of the CardioSEAL device to the delivery cable is performed with attention to a secure attachment.

prepared and loaded in a unique fashion; the reader is referred to the manufacturer's package inserts. In brief, the delivery cable and device are connected, the device is retracted into a loading tube with vigorous flushing to remove all air, and the device is loaded into the delivery catheter. The keys to optimal device preparation and loading include inspection to detect any abnormalities, verification that the attachment between the device and delivery cable is secure and capable of being unlocked, and confirmation that all air has been removed.

Delivery catheter placement and positioning

The insertion of the delivery catheter or sheath is a critical step and is guided by fluoroscopy in the anteroposterior projection. Insertion is performed as an over-the-wire technique with an extra stiff guidewire. Typically, the tip of the guidewire is placed in a left pulmonary vein for stability. The catheter is rotated gently during advancement into the right atrium to allow it to assume the typical appearance aimed at the septum. The dilator within the sheath is needed for skin entry but often is not needed to cross the PFO unless it is small or angulated. Rather, many operators intentionally remove the dilator when the tip of the catheter is in the upper IVC. This is done to flush the catheter and to minimize the chance of air entry. An alternative method is to cross the PFO with the dilator in the sheath. As the dilator is removed, there should be a continuous flushing of the sidearm of the sheath.

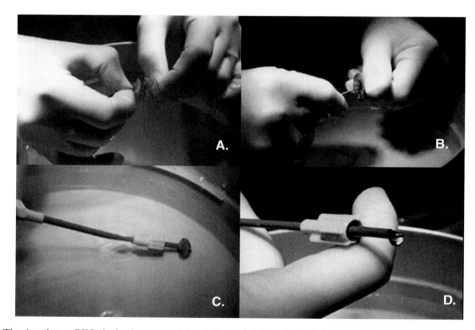

Fig. 7. The Amplatzer PFO device is prepared for delivery. (*A*) The device is inspected by separating the left and right atrial discs. (*B*) The device is screwed onto the delivery cable. (*C*) The device is pulled into the loading tube. (*D*) The device is collapsed in the loading tube and vigorous flushing finalizes the removal of all air.

Device insertion and deployment

Device delivery generally is straightforward for most PFOs. For ICE guidance, the catheter tip is deflected to the lateral wall of the right atrium and adjusted such that the entire device deployment can be observed from this parked position (Fig. 8). For both devices, the first step is insertion of the slenderized device into the delivery catheter to minimize the chance of any air entry. The next key step is the advancement of the device to the end of the delivery catheter that now is usually pulled back into the mid-left atrium. The next step is the deployment of the left atrial umbrella or disc that is achieved by pulling back on the delivery catheter and exposing the device so that it expands (Fig. 9). If the delivery catheter is too deep in the left atrium, the left atrial portion of the device will not deploy fully until the whole assembly is retracted further. Using TEE or ICE, the left atrial umbrella/disc is pulled against the PFO using gentle traction. There is slight resistance as the left atrial disc touches the left side on the atrial septum. With fluoroscopic, echocardiographic, and tactile confirmation of the correct position of the left atrial umbrella/disc, the deployment of the right atrial side of the device immediately follows by once again pulling back the delivery catheter while keeping the device–cable system fixed in space. The deployment of the right atrial portion follows and the delivery catheter is pulled back further to allow the closure device to rest in place, but still attached to the delivery cable. Final inspection of the location of the device by fluoroscopy and TEE or ICE is key. Before release

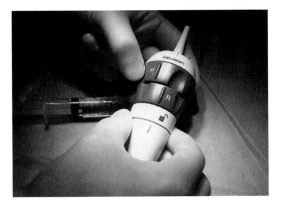

Fig. 8. The ICE catheter tip is deflected posteriorly to place the tip in the lower left aspect of the right atrium. Gentle clockwise rotation generally results in an improved image of the PFO.

of the device, it can be pushed and pulled gently to verify the correct and stable position (Fig. 10). Correct position is verified if tissue is seen between the left atrial and right atrial umbrella/disks on all sides of the PFO. Some operators use angiography rather than ultrasound for confirmation of position. Agitated saline and color-flow Doppler interrogation of PFO closure can be performed at this time; however, the device is attached to the delivery cable and this often distorts the interatrial septal anatomy to preclude an assessment of final device effectiveness in PFO closure. A gentle push and pull test of the device provides further assurance of a proper and stable device position.

Device release and assessment of device placement

The device is released per the manufacturer's instructions. Traction or excessive push on the whole assembly during the release of the device should be avoided. By either ultrasound or fluoroscopy, the release of the device is accompanied immediately by a reorientation of the device after the tethering effect of the attachment is no longer present Reorientation of the CardioSEAL device is shown (see Fig. 5C and D). The reorientation of the Amplatzer device is shown (see Fig. 9E and F). Angiography, agitated saline with ultrasound, and color-flow Doppler interrogation of PFO closure can be performed at this point. The immediate effectiveness of the device in PFO closure can be assessed best with the ultrasound bubble test using an agitated mixture of saline and a small amount of blood. This is injected directly into the delivery catheter with its tip at the IVC–right atrial junction. Valsalva maneuver should be performed with injection of bubbles immediately before the release phase. Persistent right-to-left shunting may be seen in approximately one third of patients; this usually disappears in the subsequent months in most patients, presumably as a result of device endothelialization.

Final measurements and exit of venous access

Final TEE and ICE images are acquired and the respective devices are removed. Cinefluoroscopy of the device also can be performed to document the device placement. The best projection is a cranial, LAO gantry location (see Figs. 1 and 2). We have used rotational cinefluoroscopy in a 25° cranial acquisition from 60° LAO to 60° right anterior oblique. This has replaced the need for a subsequent chest radiograph.

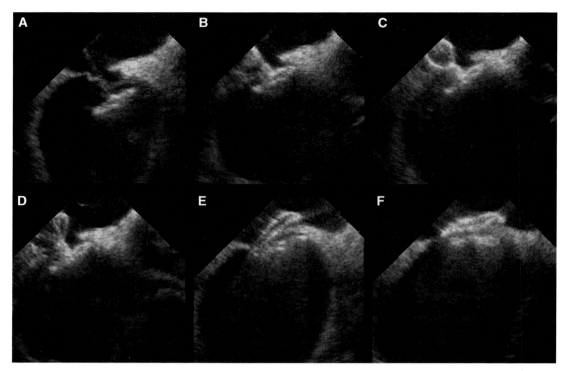

Fig. 9. These ICE images show the deployment of the Amplatzer PFO Occluder left atrium disc (*A*) Engagement of PFO. (*B*) Deployment of RA disc. (*C, D*) Final deployment position before (*E*) and after (*F*) cable release of the device.

After checking the ACT, venous sheaths typically can be removed immediately per the protocol of the cardiac catheterization laboratory. Even large venous sheaths can be removed with hemostasis within 10 minutes in the presence of moderately elevated ACT measurements. Commercially available "patches" that promote hemostasis have been used, although no data exists on their effectiveness in this setting.

Postprocedure care

There are no data on postprocedure anticoagulation or antiplatelet regimens, other than the use of aspirin for the first 6 months postprocedure. In the first 12 to 24 hours after device placement, many centers give low molecular weight heparin or unfractionated heparin at standard doses if vascular access bleeding has not

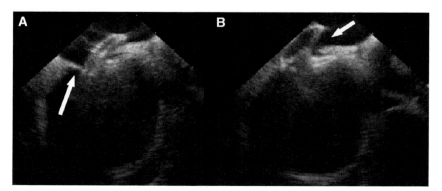

Fig. 10. The device is (*A*) pushed and (*B*) pulled to verify the correct position and stability of device placement. Tissue (*white arrows*) between the two discs should be visualized.

occurred for a reasonable period of time after sheath removal. The goals behind the use of low molecular weight heparin or unfractionated heparin are to reduce the chance of early device thrombosis and to prevent venous thrombus formation during immobilization. No randomized clinical data are available to clarify if this is best practice. Postprocedure anticoagulation is best put in the context of an individual patient. For example, patients who have hypercoagulable states that undergo PFO closure may be served best with postprocedure heparin and resumption of warfarin for some period of time. It is likely that periprocedural management issues, such as anticoagulation, will evolve into best practices as the cardiovascular community gains additional experience in PFO closure procedures; device performance; including thrombogenicity; and identification of patients who have important hypercoagulable states. It is clear that there is a low risk of any adverse events in the immediate postprocedural period. Device malfunction is exceedingly rare, bleeding is limited from the venous access, and the typical PFO closure case is a straightforward and low-risk interventional procedure, especially if ICE is used—rather than TEE—coupled with general anesthesia.

As with other venous-based procedures that use medium- to large-sized catheters, bed rest for several hours is needed initially. After documentation of hemostasis, early ambulation is possible. There seems to be no need to keep the patient's physical activity restricted.

Monitoring the patient's heart rate and rhythm probably are the most compelling reasons for an overnight hospital stay after device implantation.

Premature atrial contractions are not uncommon and have a low, but definite, chance of leading to atrial fibrillation.

It was common practice in early trials to confirm device location on the day following implantation, although many centers have discontinued this practice in uncomplicated procedures after echocardiographic and cinefluoroscopic confirmation of correct position. A plain chest radiograph or a transthoracic ultrasound may be used for this purpose. Cinefluoroscopy also can be used and takes only several minutes to perform. Newer radiograph systems with rotational capabilities allow a high-speed spin or roll acquisition that gives a three-dimensional–like assessment of device position and function.

Out-patient follow-up issues and the hand-off back to the referring physician

Important issues in patient follow-up include the routine postprocedure check, anticoagulation regimen, follow-up imaging, and monitoring for postprocedure complications. Commonly, the patient's neurologist or primary care physician can follow the patient with minimal cardiology input. The information that is communicated routinely to referring physicians after uncomplicated PFO closure are summarized in Box 6.

Some cardiologists recommend more aggressive echocardiographic follow-up. This may include a 1- and 6-month TEE with a bubble study. Some investigators believe that the 1-month study is important in detecting device thrombosis before clinical events can occur. A recent publication

---

Box 6. Postpatent foramen ovale closure communications to primary care providers

A description of the procedure, the device implanted, and the results of the early assessment of the completeness of PFO closure.

The suggested medical therapy regimen, including aspirin for 6 months for most patients and subacute bacterial endocarditis prophylaxis for 6 months.

The possible occurrence of atrial arrhythmias in the first 6 weeks.

A 6-month follow-up echocardiographic assessment with a bubble study. If the immediate postimplant bubble study was negative, this could be omitted. The 6-month study can be a transthoracic study if the preprocedure transthoracic study was of adequate quality and showed a positive bubble study. Performance of a Valsalva maneuver with a bubble test is recommended.

Any recurrent neurologic event should be evaluated aggressively and rare device thrombosis should be considered.

MRI is possible with the CardioSEAL and Amplatzer devices.

presentation showed that TEE detected device thrombus in 5% of patients [21].

Prevention, recognition, and management of unique complications of patent foramen ovale closure

Several important complications that may be seen with PFO closure may be preventable; if they occur, they require immediate recognition, evaluation, and treatment to minimize their impact. The five that are chosen for discussion include intraprocedure air embolism, device positioning problems, device embolization, postprocedure device thrombosis, and postprocedure atrial arrhythmias.

Air embolism is seen rarely during other diagnostic and therapeutic cardiac procedures. PFO closure may use large bore catheters that are placed in the left-sided circulation, in a low-pressure chamber. These conditions increase the chance of air entry into the catheter system with subsequent passage into the left atrium. Embolization of air occurs immediately with clinical manifestations that most commonly are coronary, but also can involve the central nervous system circulation.

The most common manifestation of air embolism is ST elevation on monitored electrocardiographic leads. Other manifestations of ischemia may follow immediately, including chest pain (unless the patient is under general anesthesia), sinus bradycardia, heart block, and other arrhythmias. Confusion or focal neurologic deficits may indicate embolism of air to the brain. Although permanent sequelae are rare, the rapid transition from a coherent, calm, and comfortable patient to one who has severe pain and life-threatening arrhythmia is dramatic. The duration of the ischemia is brief; improvement is apparent within a few minutes and complete resolution occurs in 5 to 10 minutes. Supplemental oxygen, analgesia, and volume expansion are general measures that may be beneficial. Treatment of arrhythmias should follow standard practices. Atropine for severe sinus bradycardia or heart block is the main medication that should be readied after the initial ST elevation is recognized. Prompt defibrillation should be available. The inferior wall location of ischemia led one group to postulate that air is most likely to enter the right coronary artery because of its more anterior location in the supine patient [22].

Some additional technical tips can minimize air embolism during the insertion of the delivery catheter or sheath. The first is the aggressive hydration of all patients and the prevention of filling pressures to be near zero in the preprocedure fasting patient. The second tip is to keep the proximal end of the delivery catheter/sheath as low as possible relative to the patient. This adds hydrostatic pressure to the column of fluid and blood in the catheter and prevents air entry. Flushing of the side port of a delivery sheath during withdrawal of the dilator is used by some cardiologists to reduce the chance of air entry during the negative pressure in the catheter that can be created by the removal of the dilator. Avoidance of catheter- and guidewire-induced coughing and subsequent creation of transient negative intrathoracic pressures also are important. Similarly, some surgeons prefer to avoid doses of sedation that produce sleeping; subsequent startling reactions with sudden deep inspiratory efforts can draw air into the delivery catheter. During advancement of the device in the delivery catheter, cinefluoroscopy can be performed briefly to see if an air bubble is being pushed ahead of the device. Air embolism remains a complication that should be minimized, if not eliminated completely, when good technique is used, the team is experienced in the procedure, and preventative measures are followed.

Device positioning problems during deployment include prolapse of a portion of the device to the incorrect side of the interatrial septum, incomplete expansion of the device, poor coadaptation of the device to the interatrial septum, and tunnel-related incomplete expansion of both sides of the device. These problems should be recognized easily with a combination of fluoroscopic and echocardiographic images during deployment. Removal of the device may be necessary. With the CardioSEAL device, it is destroyed in the process.

Device embolization is rare with PFO closure; it has been reported most commonly in the setting of large ASDs, undersized ASD devices, and in malfunction of the device-delivery cable attachment. The last was a transient problem with the Amplatzer device in late 2002 that was corrected. An example of device embolization in Fig. 11 is shown along with the technique of snare retrieval. Device embolization is more commonly into right-sided chambers, given the interatrial pressure gradient. Retrieval equipment and familiarity with retrieval techniques are necessary to have a safe and comprehensive PFO closure program. Amplatzer device may be reused after retrieval and inspection (Fig. 12).

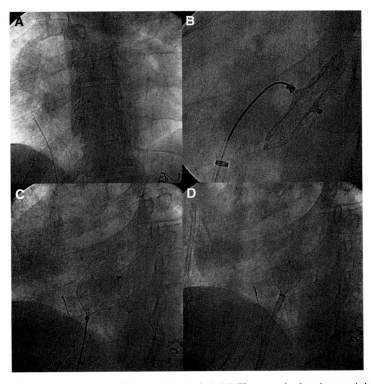

Fig. 11. (*A*) An embolized Amplatzer device (40-mm ASD device). (*B*) The snare is placed around the right atrial pin for cable attachment. (*C*) The device can be pulled into the delivery catheter and removed. (*D*) Inspection of the device should be performed before considering reinsertion.

Device thrombosis is a major complication that can lead to catastrophic events, such as embolization of thrombus, the needed for open heart surgery for device removal, and prolonged hospitalization for thrombolysis. It remains a rare and poorly understood complication. The unresolved issues include the frequency of this complication, whether underlying hypercoagulable states increase its frequency, whether the different devices have a different thrombogenicity, and whether more aggressive postimplantation anticoagulation regimens should be used routinely.

Two modes of detection of device thrombosis are typical. The first is during a routine follow-up echocardiographic study, usually a TEE study. The second is during the evaluation of a stroke in the weeks to months following implantation. Thrombi on right and left atrial sides of the device have been reported. A large and loose-appearing left-sided thrombus may prompt a surgical removal approach, whereas a right-sided thrombus may lead to a pharmacologic route of treatment. The

management of device thrombosis is similar to that of prosthetic valve thrombosis. Only isolated case studies have been reported; therefore, management remains highly individualized.

Postprocedure atrial arrhythmias occur in 3% to 4% of patients. Routine monitoring probably would detect more. Most patients who have this complication detected have symptoms that require medical attention. Palpitations and an irregular pulse are the most common symptoms. Our experience suggests that this complication occurs most commonly 4 to 6 weeks postoperatively. Other patients may have immediate postprocedure premature atrial contractions that often are asymptomatic and resolve spontaneously. The atrial arrhythmias that occur later often are symptomatic, include atrial fibrillation, and may not resolve spontaneously. Management is routine and may include β-blockers, cardioversion, or other medications to manage ventricular response and to maintain normal sinus rhythm. The key difference in the setting of post-PFO closure is

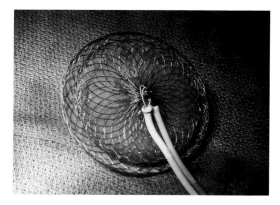

Fig. 12. This large Amplatzer ASD device was retrieved successfully using two snares that are clearly shown in this photograph. The second snare was needed to make the pin coaxial with the delivery catheter before it could be withdrawn.

that the arrhythmias likely are a transient complication that seem to resolve eventually and do not require long-term medications.

Special patient populations in patent foramen ovale closure

Patients who have hypercoagulability disorders are common in the population that is referred for PFO closure. This topic is discussed extensively elsewhere in this issue. For the PFO closure procedure, the hypercoagulability screening process has multiple important goals. First, it may increase or decrease the potential benefit from closure. Second, hypercoagulable states may increase the possibility of device thrombosis. Finally, these states may prompt the pre- and postprocedure use of heparin or low molecular weight heparin and the postprocedure use of warfarin. These issues are under intense study and the RESPECT Trial will provide insight into hypercoagulability and PFO management.

Divers may be referred for PFO closure to reduce the chance of unexplained decompression illness. Nitrogen bubbles form during normal decompression. This is termed "outgassing from peripheral tissues." In the presence of a PFO, with the additional factor of the Valsalva maneuver that often is performed intentionally by divers, there are good data to show that paradoxical embolism involves these bubbles. The finding of numerous brain lesions in divers who had large PFOs led to an appreciation in the diving community of PFO as a risk factor for decompression

illness. PFO closure has been performed in this setting.

PFO closure in the presence of an IVC filter is not rare because it is a marker of a person who has venous thromboembolic events that can become systemic events in the presence of a PFO. Performance of a percutaneous closure procedure requires a carefully considered approach. There are three possible approaches to the patient who needs percutaneous PFO closure with an IVC filter. First, the filter can be traversed using the traditional femoral venous access. Various IVC filters (eg, Greenfield [Boston Scientific, Natick, Massachusetts] and Trap-ease [Cordis Corp., Warren, New Jersey]) have been crossed successfully without dislodgment or entanglement. A more complex access is the transhepatic approach. This approach may be particularly useful in the presence of an obstructed filter or one with visible thrombus. Traditionally, interventional radiologists have performed this approach. Finally, the internal jugular approach has been used rarely with the caveat that the approach angle is challenging and special; curved delivery sheaths may be needed. Before crossing an IVC filter, it is key to evaluate its patency and whether thrombus is lodged in the filter (Fig. 13) that could be dislodged

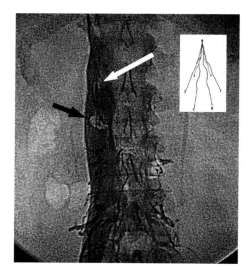

Fig. 13. A recently implanted Greenfield filter (*white arrow*) has a thrombus (*black arrow*). The patient has a large PFO and recently had a TIA and a pulmonary embolism. The inset shows the appearance of the Greenfield filter before insertion. If there was no thrombus, catheter crossing of the filter for PFO closure could have been performed safely.

and delivered into the left atrium. This can be accomplished by a preprocedure ultrasound or CT or intraprocedure angiography through a short sheath in the femoral vein. When crossing the filter, several technical tips have been suggested. A straight end-holed catheter (Goodale Lubin [USCI, Billerica, Massachusetts] or multi-purpose) should be positioned below the filter; a soft straight-tipped guidewire should be advanced carefully through the filter. After positioning the wire in the IVC–right atrial junction, exchange the end-holed catheter and short sheath with a delivery catheter that is appropriate for an Amplatzer or CardioSEAL device. The overall strategy is to minimize the number of crossings of the filter.

References

[1] Sievert H, Horvath K, Zadan E, et al. Patent foramen ovale closure in patients with transient ischemia attack/stroke. J Interv Cardiol 2001;14:261–6.

[2] Braun MU, Fassbender D, Schoen SP, et al. Transcatheter closure of patent foramen ovale in patients with cerebral ischemia. J Am Coll Cardiol 2002;39: 2019–25.

[3] Bruch L, Parsi A, Grad MO, et al. Transcatheter closure of interatrial communications for secondary prevention of paradoxical embolism: single-center experience. Circulation 2002;105:2845–8.

[4] Wahl A, Meier B, Haxel B, et al. Prognosis after percutaneous closure of patent foramen ovale for paradoxical embolism. Neurology 2001;57:1330–2.

[5] Martin F, Sanchez PL, Doherty E, et al. Percutaneous transcatheter closure of patent foramen ovale in patients with paradoxical embolism. Circulation 2002;106:1121–6.

[6] Du Z-D, Cao Q-L, Joseph A, et al. Transcatheter closure of patent foramen ovale in patients with paradoxical embolism: intermediate-term risk of recurrent neurological events. Cathet Cardiovasc Intervent 2002;55:189–94.

[7] Sievert H, Babic UU, Hausdorf G, et al on behalf of the ASDOS Study Group. Transcatheter closure of atrial septal defect and patent foramen ovale with the ASDOS device (a multi-institutional European trial). Am J Cardiol 1998;82:1405–13.

[8] Orgera MA, O'Malley PG, Taylor AJ. Secondary prevention of cerebral ischemia in patent foramen ovale: systematic review and meta-analysis. South Med J 2001;94:699–703.

[9] Mas J-L, Arquizan C, Lamy C, Zuber M, et al for the Patent Foramen Ovale and Atrial Septal Aneurysm Study Group. Recurrent cerebrovascular events associated with patent foramen ovale, atrial septal aneurysm, or both. N Engl J Med 2001;345: 1740–6.

[10] Nedeltchev K, Arnold M, Wahl A, et al. Outcome of patients with cryptogenic stroke and patent foramen ovale. J Neurol Neurosurg Psychiatry 2002;72: 347–50.

[11] DeCastro S, Cartoni D, Fiorelli M, et al. Morphological and functional characteristics of patent foramen ovale and their embolic implications. Stroke 2002;31:2407–13.

[12] Dearani JA, Ugurlu BS, Danielson GK, et al. Surgical patent foramen ovale closure for prevention of paradoxical embolism-related cerebrovascular ischemic events. Circulation 1999;100(Suppl II): II-171–5.

[13] Homma S, DiTullio MR, Sacco RL, et al. Surgical closure of patent foramen ovale in cryptogenic stroke patients. Stroke 1997;28:2376–81.

[14] Ruchat P, Bogousslavsky J, Hurni M, et al. Systematic surgical closure of patent foramen ovale in patients with cerebrovascular events due to paradoxical embolism. Early results of a preliminary study. Eur J Cardiothorac Surg 1997;11:824–7.

[15] Hagen PT, Scholz DG, Edwards WD. Incidence and size of patent foramen ovale during the first 10 decades of life: an autopsy study of 965 normal hearts. Mayo Clin Proc 1984;59:17–20.

[16] Lynch L, Schuchard G, Gross C, et al. Prevalence of right-to-left atrial shunting in a healthy population: detection by Valsalva maneuver contrast echocardiography. Am J Card 1984;53:1478–80.

[17] Chen WJ, Kuan P, Lien WP, et al. Detection of patent foramen ovale by contrast transesophageal echocardiography. Chest 1992;101:1515–20.

[18] Chenzbraun A, Pinto FJ, Schnittger I. Biplane transesophageal echocardiography in the diagnosis of patent foramen ovale. J Am Soc Echocardiogr 1993;6:417–21.

[19] Knauth M, Ries S, Pohimann S, et al. Cohort study of multiple brain lesions in sport divers: role of patent foramen ovale. BMJ 1997;314:701–5.

[20] Begin R, Gervais A, Guerin L, et al. Patent foramen ovale and hypoxemia in chronic obstructive pulmonary disease. Eur J Respir Dis 1981;62: 373–5.

[21] Krumsdorf U, Ostermayer S, Billinger K, et al. Incidence and clinical course of thrombus formation on atrial septal defect and patent foramen ovale closure devices in 1,000 consecutive patients. J Am Coll Cardiol 2004;43:302–9.

[22] Hernandez JM, Fernandez-Valls M, Vazquek de Prada JA, et al. Transient ST elevation: a finding that may be frequent in percutaneous atrial septal defect closure in adults. Rev Esp Cardiol 2002;55: 686–8.

ELSEVIER
SAUNDERS

Cardiol Clin 23 (2005) 35–45

CARDIOLOGY
CLINICS

Patent Foramen Ovale Closure: Role of the Pediatric Cardiologist

Mark Boucek, MD

*Department of Pediatrics, University of Colorado Health Sciences Center, Campus Box A036/B100,
1056 East 19th Avenue, Denver, CO 80218, USA*

History

An abnormal process of atrial septation that results in an atrial septal defect (ASD) is one of the most common cardiac abnormalities that confronts the pediatric cardiologist. An isolated ASD accounts for up to 10% of all congenital heart defects [1]. A patent foramen ovale (PFO) is not included in the incidence of ASDs. If PFOs were included in congenital heart defects, they would be the most common congenital heart defect; up to one third of children retain a potential communication from right to left atrium through a PFO. In one report, contrast echocardiographic studies demonstrated right-to-left shunting in up to 37% of children [2].

An ASD was the first lesion to be repaired surgically with open-heart techniques. An ASD also was the first intracardiac defect that was closed routinely with interventional techniques. Several devices have been developed and deployed in an ASD (see elsewhere in this issue). The diversity of devices that has been used to close an ASD has taught the interventional pediatric cardiologist much about the anatomic variations of the atrial septum. Essentially all small/moderate and many large ASDs can be closed routinely in the catheterization laboratory [3]. When ASD device technology initially was applied to adults who had a PFO, pediatric interventionalists performed most of the procedures [4]. The early experience with closing PFOs and ASDs led to the techniques that are used today. Because many patients who had complex congenital heart defects

[5] reached adulthood, the pediatric interventionalist has become involved in the care of adults. Often, a collaboration develops between adult and pediatric interventionalists to provide optimum management of complex congenital heart defects and simple defects (eg, PFO).

The adult who has a PFO usually presents for medical attention because of sequelae of a presumed paradoxic embolus across the PFO. A paradoxic embolus that causes a stroke is referred to as a cryptogenic stroke. Generally, pediatric cardiologists were not involved in caring for adults who had PFO and cryptogenic strokes until device closure became possible. As the acceptance of device closure for an ASD in children increased, the techniques and technologies were applied quickly to adults who had a PFO. The pediatric interventionalist brought vast experience with complex ASDs that needed closure and experience with the use of different types of devices [5–8]. The devices that were used to close an ASD had different design features that made them uniquely better suited to closing certain types of defects; these differences also could be important for PFO closure.

A PFO occurs as the result of failed complete septation of the atrial septum. The septation process is complex and can lead to many anatomic variants, all of which fall under the label of a PFO. If a PFO was a single characteristic defect, the experience of the pediatric interventionalist would not be required; however, the clinical entity of a PFO is not a single anatomic abnormality and the experience that is gained by the pediatric interventionalist in closing secundum ASDs may be helpful in managing the spectrum of patients who have a PFO. For example, the patient who

E-mail address: boucek.mark@tchden.org

0733-8651/05/$ - see front matter © 2005 Elsevier Inc. All rights reserved.
doi:10.1016/j.ccl.2004.10.011

has an aneurysm of the septum primum is at greatest risk for paradoxic events [9]. The aneurysmal septum primum frequently has multiple openings [10] and the morphology may influence the ability of a given device to seal the openings. Experience with devices that cover—versus fill—the primary defect may allow for device choice and placement to enhance the likelihood of complete closure. Other examples of complex anatomy exist, such as multiple defects, deficient septum secundum with superior displacement, true tunnel-like anatomy, and wedging of the aortic root into the atrial septum. These anatomic features are discussed later. Because PFO anatomy is variable, the pediatric interventionalist should continue to play a role in dealing with adults who have a PFO that needs device closure.

As we better understand the late risks that are associated with a PFO in children, it is likely that the pediatric interventionalist also may take an active role in closing PFOs in at-risk subgroups of children.

Atrial septal anatomy: developmental perspective

The atrial septum forms from three different embryologic structures: the septum primum, the septum secundum, and the endocardial cushions [11]. Only the septum primum and septum secundum contribute to the formation of the foramen ovale; if it remains open it becomes the PFO. The foramen ovale is delineated by the free edge of the septum secundum superiorly on the right side of the septum and the free edge of the perforation in the septum primum on the left side of the atrial septum (Fig. 1). The septum primum forms initially and completes septation of the atria by fusing with the endocardial cushions. An opening develops in the cephalic portion of the septum primum by an apoptotic mechanism that creates the ostium secundum. The septum secundum then develops, in part, by an infolding of the cephalic portions of the right atrial wall and grows downward to cover the ostium secundum from the right side.

Fetal hemodynamics allow shunting of blood from right atrium to left atrium through the ostium secundum by a separation of the septum secundum and septum primum—the foramen ovale (Fig. 2). After birth, hemodynamic forces close the foramen ovale and prevent left-to-right shunting. The septum primum and septum secundum are supposed to fuse in the region of the fossa ovalis to seal the atrial septum. In up to 25% of adults, however, a potential communication is left unsealed—the PFO [12].

The mechanisms that cause a PFO can be a deficiency in the septum primum or septum secundum or failure of these structures to fuse. The involvement of different embryologic structures explains the anatomic variations that are encountered in the adult who has a PFO [13]. The typical or common form of PFO is due to a failure of fusion—rather than a deficiency in septum secundum or primum—and creates the tunnel appearance (Fig. 3).

Thinning and redundancy of the septum primum creates the tissue of an atrial septal aneurysm. This aneurysmal tissue often contains multiple perforations that failed to coalesce embryologically into a single ostium secundum. The

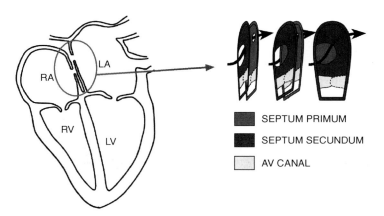

SEPTUM PRIMUM

SEPTUM SECUNDUM

AV CANAL

Fig. 1. Schematic representation of the structures leading to a PFO in the developing heart. The arrow represents flow underneath the septum secundum through the ostium secundum and into the left atrium (LA) past the septum primum. LV, left ventricle; RA, right atrium; RV, right ventricle.

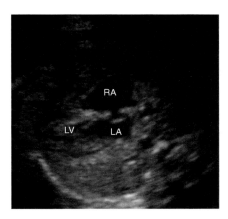

Fig. 2. Echocardiographic image of a fetal PFO. Color flow mapping shows right-to-left shunt.

aneurysmal tissue may become herniated beneath the septum secundum and allow for a communication between right and left atrium. Echocardiographically, the aneurysm of the septum primum can be seen swinging dynamically from right to left with respiratory variation (Fig. 4) [14]. It was speculated that movement of the aneurysm creates vortices and localized negative pressure that may draw thrombotic, potentially embolic material across the atrial septum.

Deficiency of the septum secundum can uncover the ostium secundum and prevent fusion of the septum primum and septum secundum. Deficiencies in the septum secundum tend to minimize the length of the tunnel of a PFO. When the septum secundum is deficient, the roof of the right atrium is in closer proximity to the PFO on the right side of the atrial septum. When the aortic root is wedged between the roof of the right and left atria and the septum secundum is deficient, the superior aspect of the right side of the PFO is closer to the aortic root (Fig. 5). Perforation of the right atrial roof by an ASD device in this scenario could result in catastrophic perforation of the aortic root. This risk of perforation may be higher for a PFO that results from a deficient septum secundum than a typical ASD because the inferior margin of the ostium secundum is more superior (cephalad); this forces the device toward the roof of the right atrium which is not protected by the septum secundum. On the left side of the septum, the superior margins of the septum primum and the roof of the left atrium are above the wedged portion of the aortic root; this makes catastrophic perforation less likely on the left side.

Occasionally, a defect in the closure of the foramen ovale can occur in conjunction with a separate ASD that is remote from the fossa ovalis (Fig. 6). Usually, these are inferior, are due to abnormalities of fusion of the septum primum to the endocardial cushions, and are called simple ostium primum type of ASD. Presence of an additional remote ASD usually requires two devices to achieve complete closure.

Patent foramen ovale in association with congenital heart disease: temporary balloon occlusion trial

The fact that a PFO is so common means that it frequently occurs with other forms of congenital

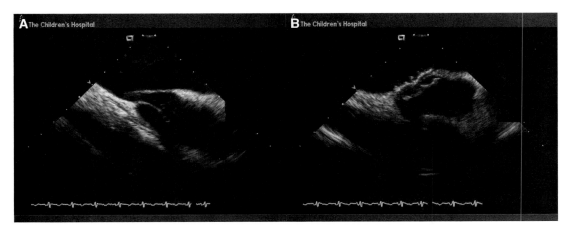

Fig. 3. (A) Intracardiac echocardiographic image demonstrating the marked overlap of the septum secundum and septum primum which creates a type of tunnel PFO. (B) With a compliant tunnel, an ASD device can realign the overlapping septae, close the PFO, and eliminate the tunnel.

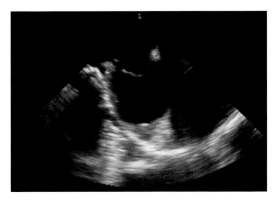

Fig. 4. Transesophageal echocardiography demonstrating prominent aneurysmal-type PFO.

heart disease. When congenital cardiac anomalies cause elevation in right-sided pressures, a PFO can allow for right-to-left shunting that causes hypoxemia. In the era of surgical repair, the PFO was closed as part of surgical correction. In the current era of interventional management, a PFO may need to be closed as part of an overall catheter intervention. A PFO also can be left open or created at the time of surgery to allow right-to-left decompression in the early postoperative period. Later, these defects can be closed with percutaneously placed devices.

Right heart structural abnormalities that can cause right-to-left atrial shunting through a PFO include pulmonic stenosis, tricuspid stenosis, tricuspid regurgitation, Ebstein's anomaly, and

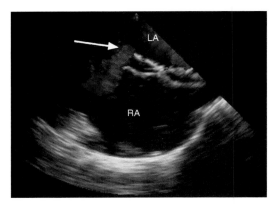

Fig. 6. Transesophageal echocardiographic image showing the presence of a separate, remote inferior simple ostium primum–type ASD. The PFO has been closed with a device. Color flow shows left-to-right shunt through the second ASD.

tetralogy of Fallot (Fig. 7). When a PFO is associated with structural heart disease, the right-to-left shunting may be hemodynamically necessary. To test whether a patient will tolerate PFO closure, balloon occlusion of the communication is performed during sizing [15]. Usually the balloon is left inflated for 5 to 10 minutes (Fig. 8). Right heart pressures, cardiac output, and saturations are recorded before and during balloon occlusion. If the right atrial pressure increases only minimally (<5 mm Hg) and if the

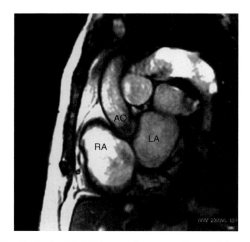

Fig. 5. Sagittal MRI image demonstrating wedging of the aortic root into the atrial septum and creating, in part, the separation between right and left atrium.

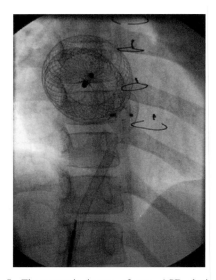

Fig. 7. Fluoroscopic image of two ASD devices in a patient who has Ebstein's malformation.

cardiac output is maintained during balloon occlusion, it generally is safe to proceed with closure of the PFO. To ensure that the balloon completely occludes the PFO, systemic saturations should increase to near normal levels. Complete balloon occlusion also should be confirmed with color Doppler and contrast echocardiography. In adults who have PFO and right ventricular dysfunction (eg, due to chronic pulmonary hypertension or ischemic heart disease), the balloon occlusion trial also may be appropriate before PFO closure. The techniques for PFO closure in this setting are similar to those described elsewhere in this issue, with the exception of the balloon occlusion trial.

When other cardiac defects occur with a PFO, closure of the PFO is delayed until surgery or interventional catheterization has been performed to deal with the primary lesion. Some complex congenital defects (eg, single ventricle) never will be repaired but may receive palliation in the form of a Fontan procedure. This procedure diverts systemic venous return directly to the pulmonary circulation and bypasses a cardiac pumping mechanism. The equivalent of a PFO can develop or be created during the Fontan procedure to help decompress the elevated right atrial pressures. When these are created at surgery (fenestrated Fontan) they usually are small (~4 mm) and aid in postoperative recovery [16]. These defects can be closed percutaneously (after trial occlusion) using techniques that are used to close PFOs [15,17]. Because they are small openings, small devices usually can be used to close the fenestration easily (Fig. 9). Right-to-left shunting can develop spontaneously in some patients who

underwent a Fontan procedure, presumably through primitive channels (eg, Thebesian system). These openings can be tortuous and not amenable to standard PFO/ASD devices, but can be closed with other types of devices (eg, patent ductus arteriosus occluder, Grifka bag, Gianturco coils).

A PFO also can complicate acquired heart disease. Following an acute myocardial infarction, changes in right and left ventricular compliance can favor right-to-left atrial shunting and "opening" of a PFO. The previously unsuspected PFO can allow right-to-left shunting in atrial diastole and cause hypoxemia [18]. The PFO also can allow left-to-right shunting in atrial systole and deprive the left ventricle of active ventricular filling; this decreases preload and impairs left ventricular stroke volume. Closing the PFO in this scenario may improve systemic oxygenation and cardiac output. This hemodynamic paradox also can effect pediatric patients adversely following open cardiac repair when an unsuspected PFO is present.

Atrial septal anatomy and the influence on device design and size

Schematically, the atrial septum appears flat and well-suited for occlusion devices. In reality, the atrial septum is a complex, three-dimensional structure. Anatomic variations in cardiac position can complicate further the approach for closure of an ASD or PFO. Furthermore, defects in the atrial septum can have complex shapes and may be asymmetric, whereas all current devices to close

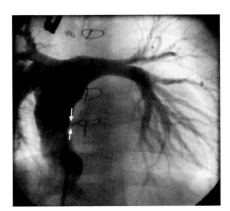

Fig. 8. Right atrial angiogram of a patient who has a fenestrated Fontan circulation and right-to-left shunting.

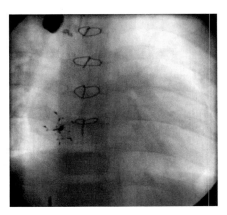

Fig. 9. Small sized ASD device occluding the fenestration (in Fig. 8) following successful trial of balloon occlusion.

ASDs are symmetric and have simple shapes. Despite the mismatch between atrial septal anatomy and the geometry of devices, they are effective in closing defects in most situations. The complications (eg, perforation, arrhythmia, local irritation, friction lesion) that result from a mismatch between anatomy and device geometry are infrequent and may be minimized by device design and size.

In patients in whom the primary defect that causes a PFO is incomplete fusion of the septum primum and septum secundum, the communication is tunnel-like. The hooding of the tunnel by the septum secundum separates the right atrial opening from the roof of the right atrium. Often, the potential size of the tunnel is much larger than the apparent size on echocardiography. This is caused by a failure to fuse over a wide area in the region of the fossa ovalis. When sizing with a static balloon, the septum secundum separates further from the septum primum to yield a larger potential size of the PFO (Figs. 3 and 10). In this situation the tissues usually are compliant. Placement of a device tends to shorten the tunnel, forces the edges of the two septae together, and effectively closes the PFO. Most sized devices will be effective in this scenario if the device design forces the two septae together to lead to fusion; however, a larger device that is appropriate to the stretched diameter of the PFO offers a margin of safety against dislodgment, particularly when considering the compliant structures of the atrial septum.

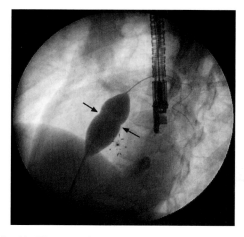

Fig. 10. Fluoroscopic recording of a sizing balloon in a small PFO which opened widely with the sizing balloon (compliant tunnel).

When the defect in fusion is only partial, the tunnel-type of PFO often is much less compliant. The semirigid tunnel can distort or deform the device that is intended to close the defect, particularly if oversized devices are used (Fig. 11). This can result in poor approximation of the device to the right or left side of the atrial septum. The device also can fail to obliterate an asymmetric tunnel completely and leave a residual right-to-left shunt. A smaller device with a small joining waist may be best suited for a semirigid tunnel PFO. Many creative approaches have been tried to overcome the limitations of this rigid tunnel anatomic variant. These approaches, such as traction on the device to help shorten the tunnel, balloon angioplasty to create a more symmetric opening, and transeptal puncture in the fossa ovalis to create a new opening that can be closed with a device that also covers the original PFO, have been used successfully to close noncompliant, tunnel-type PFOs. Many of these approaches were developed by pediatric interventionalists based on experience that was gained from creating and closing ASDs in children who had congenital heart disease [19].

Aneurysmal patent foramen ovale

An aneurysm of the septum primum that is associated with a PFO is the anatomic variant with the greatest risk of cryptogenic stroke. Often, the aneurysm has several perforations that can present a challenge for device closure. For most aneurysmal-type PFOs, it is most effective to treat the entire aneurysm as an ASD. The diameter at the base of the aneurysm—the true fossa ovalis—is the diameter to consider when choosing the device size to close the defect. The entire aneurysm is covered or compressed by the device to close the PFO and eliminate the mobile, redundant portion of the atrial septum (septum primum) (Fig. 12). When there are multiple perforations in the aneurysm, it usually is best to cross through the most central orifice; however, the tissue of the aneurysm usually is compliant and the ASD device can be effective, even when a peripheral perforation is crossed. Rarely, the aneurysm and underlying fossa ovalis is so large that a device cannot bridge the entire region of the fossa ovalis effectively. Some redundant aneurysmal tissue may remain uncovered. If the PFO and accessory perforations are closed and most of the aneurysm is stabilized under the device, it is our experience

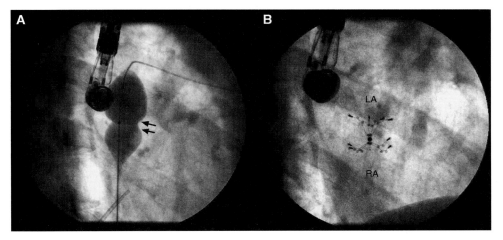

Fig. 11. (*A*) A fluoroscopic image of the sizing balloon inflated in a restrictive tunnel showing the elongated waist. (*B*) Device placement in a restrictive tunnel shows smooth apposition of the right-sided arms, whereas the left-sided arms are still distorted within the tunnel.

that the entire aneurysm will appear to be stabilized on late follow-up. In certain situations with multiple perforations in an aneurysm and a large true fossa ovalis, two devices may be required to cover the fossa and all perforations.

The aneurysmal-type PFO often can be identified in pediatric patients because it is an embryologic redundancy of the septum primum, rather than an acquired abnormality (Fig. 13). These patients should be counseled about potential risks of emboli. In high-risk situations for embolic events (eg, in-dwelling central catheters, deep vein thrombosis, long bone fractures, underwater diving), prophylactic closure of the defect may be indicated.

Catheter approach

For pragmatic reasons, pediatric interventionalists usually have approached transvenous ASD closure from the femoral vessels. The femoral venous approach is most effective because the embryologic reason for a PFO was to direct venous return from the inferior vena cava across the atrial septum to the left side of the heart. Thus, the geometry is arranged such that the course of the PFO is from inferior to superior; it is easiest to cross when the catheter is advanced from the inferior vena cava. This geometric relationship is also true in adult patients. Transhepatic approach also maintains the correct catheter alignment to the PFO.

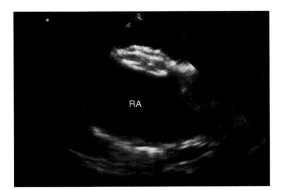

Fig. 12. Transesophageal echocardiography demonstrating the coverage of a large PFO aneurysm with the closure device.

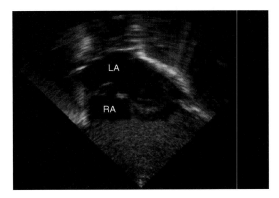

Fig. 13. Echocardiographic image of an aneurysmal atrial septum and PFO identified in a pediatric patient before any clinical events.

When the inferior vena cava approach is used, the geometry of the atrial septum is such that the plane of the atrial septum is not perpendicular to the device delivery sheath (Fig. 14). The delivery sheath and device will distort the atrial septum because of this malalignment. When the device is deployed partially, the cephalic–anterior portion of the atrial septum will approximate the edges of the device first. Further traction on the device will engage more of the atrial septum; however, the inferior portions of the device still will be separated from the inferior aspect of the ASD on the left side. When the PFO is of the noncompliant tunnel-type, a fair amount of traction can be applied that can shorten the tunnel and allow the device to approximate the left atrial side of the septum more symmetrically. If the PFO is large (stretched diameter >15 mm) or in the case of a true ASD, care must be used when bringing the device toward the left atrial side of the septum. If excessive traction is used, the superior aspect of the device may be pulled through the defect, even when the inferior aspect of the device is still away from the left side of the septum (Fig. 15).

When the left atrial side of the device is deployed completely and the superior aspect of the device is in contact correctly with the left atrial side of the septum, the right side of the device can be deployed. Imaging studies confirm that the appropriate sides of the device are on the appropriate sides of the septum. If the device position is correct, the device is released from the delivery system. When the device is released, the atrial

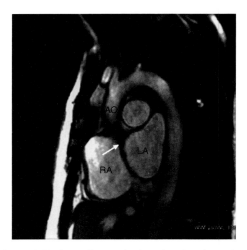

Fig. 15. MRI image in a sagittal section showing a short septum secundum which places the atrial defect superiorly and in closer approximation to the aortic root.

septum is no longer distorted and the device will reorient to the true anatomic plane of the atrial septum. Occasionally, the movements of the device with this reorientation are striking.

When there is a remote additional ASD (as in the septum primum inferiorly), a second device is necessary. When both devices are in position, the three-dimensional anatomy of the atrial septum becomes evident. The device that is placed in the true PFO may end up nearly perpendicular to an appropriately placed device in the simple primum–type ASD (Fig. 16). The complex curvilinear portions of the atrial septum occur near the edges—inferiorly toward the inferior vena cava, anteriorly where the aortic root is wedged, and superiorly near the superior vena cava and right pulmonary vein orifice. When the septum secundum is deficient, the curvilinear portions at the roof (superior or cephalic aspect of the septum) of the right side of the atrial septum can be forced against the superior aspect of an ASD device (see Fig. 15). This situation may increase the risk of perforation.

Atrial septal defect closure in pediatric patients

Several generations of devices have developed and applied to children who had an ASD. Functionally, the outcome with devices have been similar, with high closure rates [3,5,6,8]. Size, flexibility, placement, and risk of embolization have been the major benefactors of on-going device refinement [7,23]. Size of the ASD in

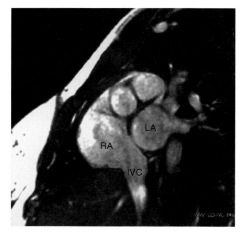

Fig. 14. MRI image in a sagittal plane showing the acute angle between the entrance of the inferior vena cava into the right atrium and the plane of the atrial septum.

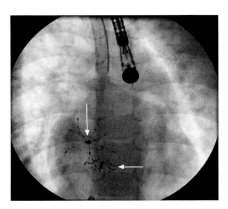

Fig. 16. Fluoroscopic image showing two devices in a PFO and a second remote ASD. The devices appear to be in different planes; this demonstrates the curvilinear nature of the atrial septum.

relation to the overall size of the atrial septum was a major limiting factor to device ASD closure in the early era. Later, centering devices that "filled" (much as the Amplatzer device; AGA Medical, Goldenvalley, Minnesota) rather than "covered," made closure of larger ASDs (up to 40 mm) feasible. Flexible devices that "cover" the ASD (Helix; WL Gore & Associates, Inc., Flagstaff, Arizona) are in trials and may be suited better for the eccentric ASD near the curvilinear margins of the atrial septum.

The frontier in ASD closure involves the large ASD that extends to the margin of the atrial septum. These defects lack a rim of tissue around the hole. As the percentage of the defect without rim increases, the concern about device stability increases. If more than 90° is without sufficient rim, it is extremely difficult to seat a device properly. Commonly, the deficiency in ASD rim occurs in the region of the wedged aortic root. Preformed catheters, such as the Hausdorf (Cook Group Inc., Bloomington, Indiana) can reorient device deployment posteriorly; this allows the device to be engaged on the left side without pulling through the region of deficient rim anteriorly near the aortic root.

When there is a deficiency of the ASD rim, the tendency has been to oversize the device to ensure stability. The oversized device tends to create a rim by pinching tissue at the atrial wall or aortic root. The safe limits of the combination of ASD size, rim deficiency, and device oversizing are being defined and may vary with device and ASD location.

Effectiveness of patent foramen ovale device closure

Reported rates of PFO closure using a percutaneous device are approximately 90% [5–8]. Residual atrial septal communications usually are due to unrecognized additional septal defects or inadequate device contact with the atrial septal surface in semirigid, tunnel-type PFOs. An appreciation of atrial septal embryogenesis and morphology can guide the choice and size of a device to optimize complete closure of the PFO. Recurrent embolic events were associated with residual defects in some patients [20,21]. Although in most patients who have contrast echocardiography evidence of a residual opening, the effective orifice is so small that significant emboli usually are excluded. In our series of 100 consecutive patients who had a PFO, complete closure was obtained in 96 patients; there were no recurrent strokes within 2 years of follow-up. These results are similar to published series [22]. One patient had one episode of a presumed transient ischemic attack that occurred within 3 months after PFO closure. Thus, device closure usually is effective at closing a PFO and markedly reduces the recurrence rate of cryptogenic stroke [23,24].

Risks of patent foramen ovale closure

The risks of device closure of PFO are small. Rarely, significant morbidity can occur [24]. Embolic events that occur during device placement have been reported. The large sheaths that are used for device delivery make air emboli a constant concern that probably cannot be eliminated completely. In our series of 100 consecutive patients who had PFO, two episodes of air emboli were observed with transient S-T segment changes. Exuberant thrombosis on the PFO device has been described rarely. Most patients who are referred for PFO closure have been screened for abnormalities that could increase the risk of excessive clot forming on the device; however, the exact causes of excess device thrombosis are unknown. Pediatric interventionalists routinely anticoagulate with heparin and maintain an activated clotting time of approximately 250 seconds or greater. Antiplatelet therapy has not been used routinely during the procedure. This strategy has resulted in minimizing thrombotic and hemorrhagic complications to the point that they are reportable. Erosion of the atrial wall by a PFO device also is extremely rare; however, because of the catastrophic potential of atrial wall erosion, there is an ongoing effort to match the PFO anatomy to the closure device. Current imaging techniques may be inadequate at defining patients who are at risk for device perforation and there has been interest in three-dimensional reconstruction techniques. MRI and echocardiography have been used to define three-dimensional atrial septal anatomy. For the typical PFO, the relationship of the PFO to the roof of the atria may be most critical in preventing postprocedural perforations. A deficient secundum septum can be used as a guide for those who may be at risk.

Procedural cardiac perforations also are infrequent unless the transeptal puncture approach is used for tunnel-like PFOs [25]. Infectious risk is minimized by a sterile environment and routine use of prophylactic antibiotic coverage. Thus, the overall risks of PFO closure should be low (<1%) and justify the percutaneous approach as the technique of choice. The experience of pediatric interventionalists may help to minimize risk in situations of complex atrial septal anatomy or multiple ASDs. Current imaging techniques, including multi-plane transesophageal echocardiography, cannot identify all patients who have complicated PFO anatomy and the advantages of three-dimensional reconstruction have not been defined fully.

Summary and future role of pediatric interventionalists in closure of patent foramen ovale

Although a PFO is a developmental defect, it traditionally has not been considered to be significant in children. Thus, therapy for a PFO usually has been performed in adults. Patients who have cryptogenic strokes are seen by adult neurologists and referred primarily to adult cardiologists. Pediatric interventionalists were involved in PFO closure because they were associated intimately with the development of devices to close ASDs in children. Pediatric interventionalists also are in the unique position of creating an opening between right and left atrium equivalent to a PFO [26]. These created PFOs may need to be closed at a later date. Because these devices are still in development and likely will find application to adults who have PFOs, the pediatric interventionalist should continue to play a significant role in PFO closure in children and adults. Closure of complex PFO anatomy also may use the experience of pediatric

cardiologists. Collaboration between pediatric and adult cardiologists provides the optimum arrangement, although pragmatically, it is difficult at times. Perhaps as the volume of PFO closures increases, the logistics of a collaborative arrangement will ease. Additionally, the pragmatics of stocking the necessary catheters, devices, and retrieval systems make a collaborative arrangement more attractive. Finally, the imaging requirements to assess anatomy preclosure and evaluate device position at the time of closure should encourage a closer working relationship between pediatric and adult cardiologists in general.

References

[1] Beerman LB, Zuberbulher FR. Atrial septal defect. Pediatr Cardiol 1987;1:541–62.
[2] Van Hare GF, Silverman NH. Contrast two-dimensional echocardiography in congenital heart disease: techniques, indications and clinical utility. J Am Coll Cardiol 1989;13:673–86.
[3] Magee AG, Qureshi SA. Closure of atrial septal defects by transcatheter devices. Pediatr Cardiol 1997;18:326–7.
[4] Bridges ND, Hellenbrand W, Latson L, et al. Transcatheter closure of patent foramen ovale after presumed paradoxical embolism. Circulation 1992;86:1902–8.
[5] Sievert H, Babic UU, Hausdorf G, et al. Transcatheter closure of atrial septal defect and patent foramen ovale with ASDOS device (a multi-institutional European trial). Am J Cardiol 1998;82:1405–13.
[6] Rao PS, Sideris EB, Hausdorf G, et al. International experience with secundum atrial septal defect occlusion by the buttoned device. Am Heart J 1994;128:1022–35.
[7] Kaulitz R, Paul T, Hausdorf G. Extending the limits of transcatheter closure of atrial septal defects with the double umbrella device (CardioSEAL). Heart 1998;80:54–9.
[8] Masura J, Gavora P, Formanek A, et al. Transcatheter closure of secundum atrial septal defects using the new self-centering Amplatzer septal occluder: initial human experience. Cathet Cardiovasc Diagn 1997;42:388–93.
[9] Mügge A, Daniel WG, Angermann C, et al. Atrial aneurysm in adult patients. A multicenter study using transthoracic and transesophageal echocardiography. Circulation 1995;91:2785–92.
[10] Ewert P, Berger F, Vogel IM, et al. Morphology of perforated atrial septal aneurysm suitable for closure by transcatheter device placement. Heart 2000;84:327–31.

[11] Valdes-Cruz LM, Cayre RO. Echocardiographic diagnosis of congenital heart disease. Philadelphia: Lippincott-Raven Publishers; 1999.

[12] Meissner I, Whisnant JP, Khandheria BK, et al. Prevalence of potential risk factors for stroke assessed by transesophageal echocardiography and carotid ultrasonography: The SPARC Study. Mayo Clin Proc 1999;74:862–9.

[13] Marshal AC, Lock JE. Structural and compliant anatomy of the patent foramen ovale in patients undergoing transcatheter closure. Am Heart J 2000;140:303–7.

[14] Cabanes L, Mas JL, Cohen A, et al. Atrial septal aneurysm and patent foramen ovale as risk factors for cryptogenic stroke in patients less than 55 years of age: a study using transesophageal echocardiography. Stroke 1993;24:1865–73.

[15] Senzaki H, Naito C, Masutani S, et al. Hemodynamic evaluation for closing interatrial communication after fenestrated Fontan operation. J Thorac Cardiovasc Surg 2001;121(6):1200–2.

[16] Lemler MS, Scott WA, Leonard SR, et al. Fenestration improves clinical outcome of the fontan procedure: a prospective, randomized study. Circulation 2002;105(2):207–12.

[17] Goff DA, Blume ED, Gauvreau K, et al. Clinical outcome of fenestrated Fontan patients after closure: the first 10 years. Circulation 2000;102(17):2094–9.

[18] Silver MT, Lieberman EH, Thibault GE. Refractory hypoxemia in inferior myocardial infarction from right-to-left shunting through a patent foramen ovale: a case report and review of the literature. Clin Cardiol 1994;17:627–30.

[19] Ruiz CE, Alboliras ET, Pophal SG. The puncture technique: a new method for transcatheter closure of patent foramen ovale. Cathet Cardiovasc Intervent 2001;53:369–72.

[20] Hung J, Landzberg MG, Jenkins KJ, et al. Closure of patent foramen ovale for paradoxical emboli: intermediate-term risk of recurrent neurological events following transcatheter device placement. J Am Coll Cardiol 2000;35(5):1311–6.

[21] Windecker S, Wahl A, Chatterjee T, et al. Percutaneous closure of patent foramen ovale in patients with paradoxical embolism: long-term risk of recurrent thromboembolic events. Circulation 2000;101:893–8.

[22] Martin F, Sanchez PL, Doherty E, et al. Percutaneous transcatheter closure of patent foramen ovale in patients with paradoxical embolism. Circulation 2002;106:1121–6.

[23] Sievert H. Interventional versus surgical closure of atrial and ventricular septal defects: advantages and limitations of the catheter-base approach. J Intervent Cardiol 2000;13:493–501.

[24] Wahl A, Meier B, Haxel B, et al. Prognosis after percutaneous closure of patent foramen ovale for paradoxical embolism. Neurology 2001;57:1330–2.

[25] Trepels T, Zeplin H, Sievert H, et al. Cardiac perforation following transcatheter PFO closure. Cathet Cardiovasc Intervent 2003;58:111–3.

[26] Chatrath R, Cabalka AK, Driscoll DJ, et al. Fenestrated Amplatzer device for percutaneous creation of interatrial communication in patients after Fontan operation. Catheter Cardiovasc Interv 2003;60(1):88–93.

ELSEVIER
SAUNDERS

Cardiol Clin 23 (2005) 47–52

CARDIOLOGY
CLINICS

The Echocardiographer and the Diagnosis of Patent Foramen Ovale

Edward A. Gill, Jr, MD[a,c,*], Robert A. Quaife, MD[b]

[a]Division of Cardiology, Department of Medicine, University of Washington School of Medicine,
1959 Pacific Avenue NE, Seattle, WA 98195, USA
[b]Division of Cardiology, Department of Medicine, University of Colorado Health Sciences Center,
4200 East Ninth Avenue, Box B120, Denver, Colorado 80262, USA
[c]Harborview Medical Center, 325 Ninth Avenue, Seattle, WA 98104, USA

Echocardiography is the mainstay for the diagnosis of patent foramen ovale (PFO). From a clinical standpoint, PFO should be suspected in any patient who has a cryptogenic stroke, especially in a patient who is younger than 55 years of age who has a history of cryptogenic stroke. The suspicion should be particularly high when additional clinical factors accompany the stroke. Examples include the presence of a deep venous thrombosis in the setting of a stroke, although deep venous thrombosis rarely is confirmed in the setting of PFO and stroke. A second example is a stroke that occurs while straining or performing the Valsalva maneuver (eg, while having a bowel movement). These are classic examples of a stroke that is caused by a paradoxic embolus.

If the clinical suspicion is high, a high-quality echocardiogram is indicated—in most instances to include saline contrast echocardiography. When sending a patient for an echocardiogram to diagnose PFO, it is important to refer to an echocardiography laboratory that has experience in making this diagnosis. Experience is found in echocardiography laboratories that perform high volumes of studies specifically for the diagnosis of stroke and perform contrast studies for this purpose. In addition, seeking out an echocardiography laboratory that is accredited is advised.

Role of traditional methods of shunt detection

Generally, traditional methods of shunt detection (eg, oximetry, indocyanine green curves) are not useful for the detection of PFO because the degree of shunt is too minute [1]. Oximetry requires detection of arterial stepup or stepdown. In the setting of PFO, it would require a stepdown from the pulmonary vein oxygen saturation to the left atrial saturation. There are occasional cases of patients who have desaturation from a PFO.

Role of transthoracic echocardiography

The initial screening for PFO and interatrial septal communication, in general, is done with transthoracic color Doppler and spectral Doppler (Fig. 1). This is followed by a saline contrast study. The saline contrast study must be done with exquisite detail to enhance the sensitivity of the examination. First, the saline contrast must be performed with the correct type of saline. Regular normal saline from a typical hospital intravenous solution will not work nearly as well as the specially bottled saline that contains benzyl alcohol as a preservative (Fig. 2). The benzyl alcohol keeps the bubbles in solution longer. Next, the contrast examination must be performed in a resting condition, and if negative, performed with Valsalva maneuver or cough. Typically, the apical views are the best for visualization. This is because in the parasternal view, injection of contrast fills the right side of the heart; this obscures the left side of the heart (Fig. 3). A contrast examination looks for the passage of contrast from the right side to the left

* Corresponding author.
E-mail address: eagill@u.washington.edu (E.A. Gill).

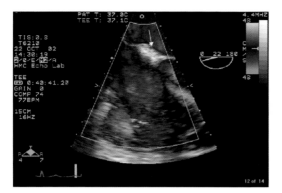

Fig. 1. The interatrial septum is imaged with color flow Doppler. This example shows a patent foramen ovale with right-to-left shunting seen by color Doppler (*arrow*). Note the small amount of shunting.

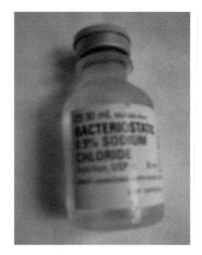

Fig. 2. Saline with benyzl alcohol.

side at the atrial level, which is consistent with PFO (Figs. 4 and 5). An important premise to saline contrast echocardiography is that the microbubbles that are created by the agitation of saline are too large (typically greater than 10μ) to pass through the pulmonary circulation. Another important detail is that contrast should appear in the left heart within three cardiac cycles. In unusual instances however, right to left intracardiac shunting still could be present after three cardiac cycles. One example would be poor cardiac output, particularly involving the right heart. Another example would be the requirement of a maneuver, either deep inspiration, Valsalva, or cough to drive contrast across the septum and this might take more than three cycles. However, in most cases when

contrast appears in the left heart in greater than three cycles, the contrast has passed through the pulmonary circuit and therefore this represents intrapulmonary rather than intracardiac shunting. Damage to the pulmonary vasculature, as occurs in the hepatopulmonary syndrome, would result in such an intrapulmonary shunt. This is present in patients who have end-stage liver disease with an accompanying pulmonary vascular component.

Having the patient cough during the saline injection is another method (in addition to the Valsalva maneuver) that increases the sensitivity of the test [2]. This is because coughing preferentially increases right atrial pressure; however, a shunt

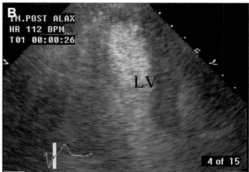

Fig. 3. (*A*) The difficulty with injecting contrast in the parasternal long axis view by echocardiography. The contrast is seen initially in the right ventricle. Because the right ventricle is between the transducer and the left ventricle (LV), the contrast shadows the view of the LV and makes it difficult to assess whether there are any bubbles in the left side of the heart. (*B*) To overcome this limitation, the apical long axis view can be used to show the same left ventricular anatomy while avoiding the shadowing. In this case, the transducer initially penetrates the LV apex rather than the right ventricle.

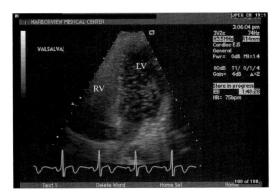

Fig. 4. Transthoracic echocardiography of a positive bubble study showing contrast present in the left ventricle. The contrast initially appears in the right ventricle.

that is detected at rest may represent a higher risk of embolization than a shunt that is produced in response to maneuvers [5]. Finally, injection of saline through the femoral vein has a greater sensitivity for detection of PFO than an injection through an antecubital vein. This is because flow through the inferior vena cava has a more direct route through a PFO than flow through the superior vena cava [3,4]. From a practical standpoint, however, it is difficult to justify placement of the intravenous line in the femoral vein, although a vein in the foot could be justified. In our echocardiography laboratory, an intravenous line is started in the foot for the evaluation of a PFO, except in patients who already have an intravenous line in place.

Although transesophageal echocardiography (TEE) has been considered to be the gold standard for the diagnosis of PFO, much of the purported superiority of TEE compared with transthoracic

echocardiography (TTE) is supported by outdated technology. Until recently, the only study that compared TTE with TEE was limited to 38 patients; nonharmonic imaging was performed using Hewlett-Packard (Andover, Massachusetts) Sonos 500 or 1500 systems. These systems use 1993 technology (and older) and were developed before the existence of harmonic imaging. This study showed a sensitivity of 50% for transthoracic contrast echocardiography [6]. Using more up-to-date technology, transthoracic contrast echocardiography was shown to have a sensitivity of 63% and specificity of 100% when using TEE as the gold standard [7]. The enhanced sensitivity was due to the addition of harmonic imaging (Fig. 6). The authors' opinion is that the echocardiographer can screen out most patients that likely cannot be diagnosed by TTE and suggest TEE in these patients. An exception would be that suspicion for PFO remains high even after a negative TTE. A particularly important point is that TTE has the advantage of being able to perform Valsalva maneuver and cough while performing imaging. These maneuvers clearly increase the sensitivity of the examination. Although it is possible to perform cough during TEE, the effort put forth by the patient often is reduced because s/he is sedated.

Role of transesophageal echocardiography

TEE should be considered when the TTE does not show a PFO, but clinical suspicion remains high; however, a good quality TTE with contrast should exclude a PFO with similar predictive value as TEE. This is particularly true with contemporary ultrasound systems that use harmonic imaging to enhance image quality; in some cases, the images are nearly indistinguishable from TEE images. Despite this statement, this has not

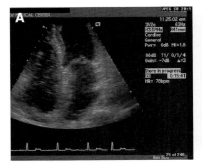
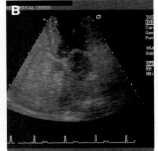
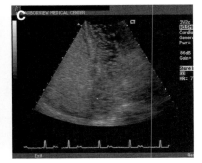

Fig. 5. Transthoracic echocardiography example of a positive bubble study showing agitated saline contrast initially present in the right heart (A), then in the right heart and left atrium (B), and finally in the left ventricle as well (C).

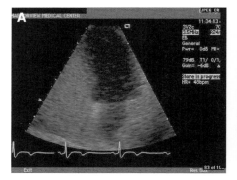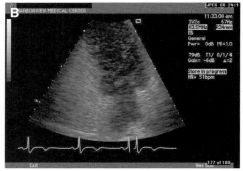

Fig. 6. Fundamental (nonharmonic) imaging of contrast (*A*) compared with harmonic imaging (*B*). Note the enhancement of the bubbles with harmonic imaging.

been confirmed in the literature. Patients who have a borderline quality TTE should seek a higher yield with the addition of TEE. Other benefits of TEE include improved visualization of the foramen ovale orifice, the ostium secundum (Fig. 7), and the interatrial septum, as well as the evaluation for atrial septal aneurysm. Atrial septal aneurysm is defined as a highly mobile septum with 1.5 cm of total medial lateral movement, 1.5 cm of movement from the midline, or a total length of the septum with significant movement of 1.5 cm (Fig. 8).

Although the evaluation ends if a PFO is excluded, if a PFO is found, further evaluation is warranted by TEE. The degree of shunt should be evaluated semiquantitatively based on the number of bubbles passing right to left and the visual size of the defect. Hence, a mild degree of shunting would be described as passage of less than five bubbles from right to left. Passage of 5-25 bubbles would be described as a moderate degree of shunting.

Greater than 25 bubbles is marked shunting (Fig. 9). Although this clearly is semiquantitative, some literature suggests that the degree of shunting correlates with the risk of recurrent stroke [8–12]. This semiquantitative method is based on previous studies that quantified shunting based on the number of contrast bubbles passing into the left atrium. In one study, after 25 bubbles or more were seen in the left atrium, the bubble count was counted as 25. This clearly did not give adequate weight to the cases [13]. In some instances, a semi-quantitative estimate of the size of the PFO can be made on the basis of the actual image (ie, how large the opening appears) [10–12]. Sometimes the open-ing can be visualized well and measured. In most cases, the opening is not visualized well; the size of the PFO only can be inferred based on the semi-quantitative nature of the contrast passing through the defect. In some studies, the presence of a Chiari network implied a greater risk of stroke due to greater degree of shunting [11] (Fig. 10).

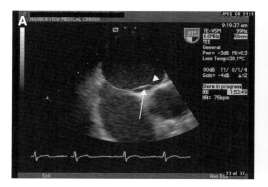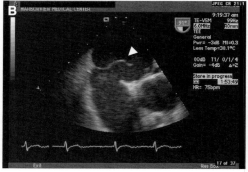

Fig. 7. Transesophageal image of a PFO that largely is closed, but with a prominent tunnel (*arrow*) and the opening of the ostium secundum (*arrowhead*) (*A*) and open, showing the septum primum (*arrowhead*) (*B*).

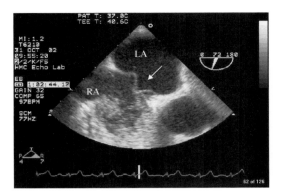

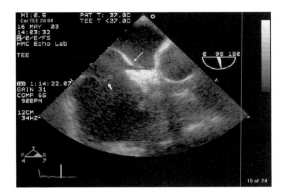

Fig. 8. Transesophageal echocardiography of a patient who has a highly aneurysmal interatrial septum (*arrow*).

Three-dimensional echocardiography

Three-dimensional (3D) echocardiography has been useful for the quantitation of size and shape of atrial septal defects. Use of 3D echocardiography has been limited for evaluation of PFO because the defect in the septum is typically small (often 1-2 mm or less) and is not within the range of resolution of 3D echocardiography. In addition, the defect is dynamic, and often only seen with maneuvers like the Valsalva maneuver, making capture of the defect difficult for 3D echocardiography. For larger defects and those with fenestrations, 3D echocardiography can be helpful. Three-dimensional echocardiography also is useful for planning the closure of septal defects and the evaluation of the closure devices after they are in place [14].

Other, competing imaging modalities

Echocardiography is the only imaging technique that has the potential to visualize the PFO.

Fig. 10. A patient who has resting hypoxia. Noncontrast image shows atrial septal aneurysm (*long arrow*) and Chiari network (*short arrow*). This patient's oxygen saturation was in the high 70% range on room air and required 50% oxygen to attain an oxygen saturation that was greater than 90%.

Contrast angiography can localize the defect if shunting is severe enough to visualize the passage of contrast through the septum; however, it cannot show the details of the septum primum and septum secundum like echocardiography. MRI has advanced rapidly and can visualize the interatrial septum; however, the fossa ovalis is not well-visualized.

Summary

PFO is diagnosed by echocardiography using the combination of transthoracic two-dimensional imaging of the interatrial septum, followed by color and spectral Doppler (and if necessary saline contrast) imaging. Transesophageal imaging is an

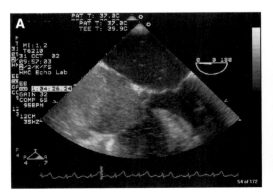

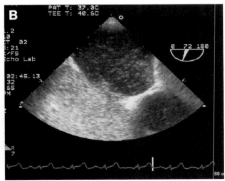

Fig. 9. Example of qualitative grading of the degree of shunt. (*A*) A few microbubbles are seen crossing to the left atrium, which is indicative of a small shunt. (*B*) A moderate degree of shunting is demonstrated with more bubbles seen in the left atrium.

important adjunct when transthoracic imaging is not conclusive or yields suboptimal images. Three-dimensional echocardiography is useful for defining fenestrations within a PFO.

References

[1] Boehrer JD, Lange RA, Willard JE, et al. Advantages and limitations of methods to detect, localize, and quantitate intracardiac right-to-left and bi-directional shunting. Am Heart J 1993;125:215–20.

[2] Stoddard MF, Keedy DL, Dawkins PR. The cough test is superior to the Valsalva maneuver in the delineation of right-to-left shunting through a patent foramen ovale during contrast transesophageal echocardiography. Am Heart J 1993;125(1):185–9.

[3] Gin KG, Huckell VF, Pollick C. Femoral vein delivery of contrast medium enhances transthoracic echocardiographic detection of patent foramen ovale. J Am Coll Cardiol 1993;22(7):1994–2000.

[4] Hamann GF, Schatzer-Klotz D, Frohlig G, et al. Femoral injection of echo contrast medium may increase the sensitivity of testing for a patent foramen ovale. Neurology 1998;50:1423–8.

[5] De Castro S, Cartoni D, Fiorelli M, et al. Morphological and functional characteristics of patent foramen ovale and their embolic implications. Stroke 2000;31:2407–13.

[6] Belkin RN, Pollack BD, Ruggiero ML, et al. Comparison of transesophageal and transthoracic echocardiography with contrast and color flow Doppler in the detection of patent foramen ovale. Am Heart J 1994;128:520–5.

[7] Ha JW, Shin MS, Kang S, et al. Enhanced detection of right-to-left shunt through patent foramen ovale by transthoracic contrast echocardiography using harmonic imaging. Am J Cardiol 2001;87: 669–71.

[8] Steiner MM, Di Tullio M, Rundek T, et al. Patent foramen ovale size and embolic brain imaging findings among patients with ischemic stroke. Stroke 1998;29:944–8.

[9] Schuchlenz HW, Weihs W, Beitzke A, et al. Transesophageal echocardiography for quantifying size of patent foramen ovale in patients with cryptogenic cerebrovascular events. Stroke 2002;33:293–6.

[10] Schuchlenz HW, Weihs W, Horner S, et al. The association between the diameter of a patent foramen ovale and the risk of embolic cerebrovascular events. Am J Med 2000;109:456–62.

[11] Kerut EK, Norfleet WT, Plotnick GD, et al. Patent foramen ovale: a review of associated conditions and the impact of physiologic size. J Am Coll Cardiol 2001;38:613–23.

[12] Kerr AJ, Buck T, Chia K, et al. Transmitral Doppler: a new transthoracic contrast method for patent foramen ovale detection and quantification. J Am Coll Cardiol 2000;35:1959–66.

[13] Homma S, DiTullio MR, Sacco RL, et al. Characteristics of patent foramen ovale associated with cryptogenic stroke. A biplane transesophageal echocardiographic study. Stroke 1994;25:582–6.

[14] Acar P, Saliba Z, Bonhoeffer P, et al. Assessment of the geometric profile of the Amplatzer and Cardioseal septal occluders by three-dimensional echocardiography. Heart 2001;85:451–3.

ELSEVIER
SAUNDERS

Cardiol Clin 23 (2005) 53–64

CARDIOLOGY
CLINICS

The Echocardiographer's role During the Placement of Patent Foramen Ovale Closure Devices

Edward A. Gill, Jr, MD[a],*, Robert A. Quaife, MD[b],
Steven L. Goldberg, MD[c]

[a]Department of Medicine, Division of Cardiology, University of Washington School of Medicine,
Harborview Medical Center, 325 Ninth Avenue, Seattle, WA 98104-9747, USA
[b]Department of Medicine, University of Colorado, 1959 Pacific Avenue NE, Box 356115, Seattle, WA 98195, USA
[c]Division of Cardiology, University of Washington School of Medicine, Harborview Medical Center,
325 Ninth Avenue, Seattle, WA 98104-9747, USA

In 2001, the US Food and Drug Administration approved the use of septal occluder devices for closing atrial septal defects and patent foramen ovale (PFO). Soon, many tertiary centers began to implant the devices. The use of these devices has resulted in a unique role for the echocardiographer. The physician, echocardiographer, and sonographer often spend a significant amount of time in the cardiac catheterization laboratory assisting the interventional cardiologist with placement of these devices [1]. The "guidance" for these devices is changing rapidly; just 2 years ago, most of these cases used transesophageal echocardiography (TEE) as the "guider." The disadvantage that TEE presents as the guiding ultrasound technique is that general anesthesia usually is used. Although TEE guidance can be performed with conscious sedation throughout a catheterization procedure, it is cumbersome for the echocardiographer and uncomfortable for the patient [2]. This is the reason that there has been a movement toward the use of intracardiac echocardiography (ICE) as the guiding technology. With access for ICE obtained through the femoral vein, the major advantage is that the interventionalist can steer the catheter (with the echocardiographer or sonographer initially aiding); general anesthesia is avoided. Our interventionalist has become the local expert with ICE and the role of the echocardiographer is

obviated. Nevertheless, TEE continues to play a significant role in the diagnostic assessment of septal defects before closure. In complicated cases, TEE is preferable to ICE during deployment of the device. With experience, however, most defects can be closed using ICE as the guidance [3].

In addition to ICE, three-dimensional (3D) echocardiography is the other emerging technology that is useful for planning closure of the atrial septal defect and for evaluation after closure. 3D echocardiography has been difficult to use as a standard adjunct during deployment of septal occluders because of the need to perform computer generated reconstruction of the images before they can be viewed. Although, 3D echocardiography can add additional information for planning closure, it is not useful during the procedure because of the time that is involved for computer reconstruction. The recent development of real-time 3D echocardiography means that this technology will have an adjunctive role in the placement of septal occluder devices. It remains to be seen whether the resolution of real-time 3D echocardiography can be enhanced to allow its general use and potential replacement of ICE.

General approach to echocardiography for the guidance of patent foramen ovale and atrial septal defect closure

The use of echocardiography for septal occluder devices can be divided into two parts: (1)

* Corresponding author.
E-mail address: eagill@u.washington.edu (E.A. Gill).

0733-8651/05/$ - see front matter © 2005 Elsevier Inc. All rights reserved.
doi:10.1016/j.ccl.2004.10.009

cardiology.theclinics.com

use for diagnosis and planning of the procedure and (2) use during the procedure. Echocardiography plays a major role in the placement of these devices from the perspective of guiding the placement and deployment of the device as well as avoiding impingement on adjacent structures. More specifically, the septal occluder devices have the potential to affect the function of the mitral and tricuspid valves and could interfere with flow in the pulmonary veins, particularly the right upper pulmonary vein, and the superior vena cava and coronary sinus. Therefore, interrogation of these structures before and after placement of the occluder device is mandatory.

Transesophageal echocardiography

TEE should be performed before virtually all atrial septal defect (ASD) and PFO closures. Only with TEE can the interatrial septum be evaluated completely for additional defects and fenestrations in the atrial septum, as well as for the anatomic variations that are present in the adjacent structures. For evaluation of PFO anatomy specifically, only TEE allows detailed evaluation of the septum primum, the foramen ovale, and the ostium secundum. Also, the sensitivity of TEE for PFO is greater, in general, than transthoracic echocardiography (TTE). The interatrial septum is best evaluated from the high esophageal view. Adjacent structures that are in close relationship to the interatrial septum that must be evaluated to avoid impingement by the device include the coronary sinus, the inferior vena cava, the superior vena cava, and the pulmonary veins, particularly the right upper and left upper pulmonary veins.

Pertinent views to obtain with transesophageal echocardiography for planning device closure

Bicaval view

The bicaval view, obtained by placing the TEE high in the esophagus with the multi-plane angle placed at roughly 110° with rightward or clockwise rotation, is useful to visualize the distance between the defect in the septum and the superior and inferior vena cava. This also is an ideal view to inject saline for the evaluation of interatrial shunting (Fig. 1).

Pulmonary veins

Typically, the pulmonary veins can be evaluated by obtaining a classic view of the aortic valve in short axis (Figs. 2 and 3) and then rotating the

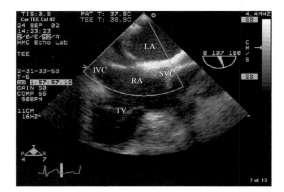

Fig. 1. Bicaval view. IVC, inferior vena cava; LA, left atrium; RA, right atrium; SVC, superior vena cava; TV, tricuspid valve.

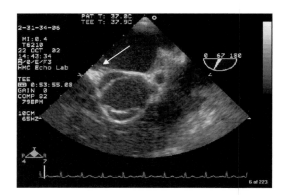

Fig. 2. The aortic valve is shown in short axis in this high esophageal view. The aortic valve is partially open in this view showing all three cusps. The flap of the patent foramen ovale is just adjacent to the aortic valve (*arrow*).

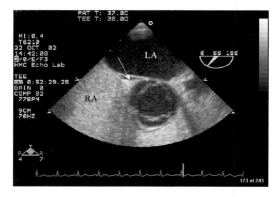

Fig. 3. The aortic valve is shown. With the addition of contrast to the right atrium, the foramen ovale and its tunnel are shown well (*arrow*).

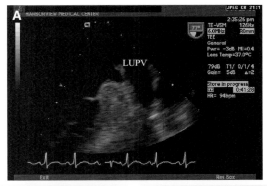

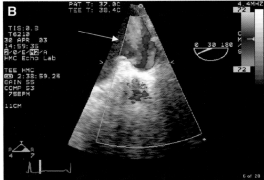

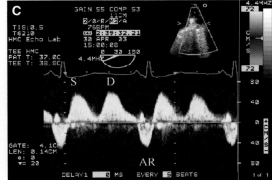

Fig. 4. In this high esophageal view, TEE shows the left upper pulmonary vein (LUPV). LSPV shown in 2D (*A*), imaged by color Doppler (*B*) and spectral pulsed Doppler (*C*). The systolic (S), diastolic (D), and atrial reversal (AR) components are shown.

probe leftward or counterclockwise toward the atrial appendage. The left upper and left lower pulmonary veins can be imaged from this position (Figs. 4 and 5). Likewise, the right upper and right lower pulmonary veins typically are obtained by marked clockwise or right rotation from a similar level, again using the short axis of the aortic valve as a starting point. Typically, the short axis view of the aortic valve is in the midesophageal view with the multi-plane angle

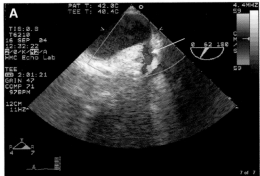

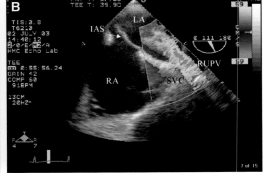

Fig. 5. (*A*) This high esophageal view by TEE shows the left lower pulmonary vein. The left lower pulmonary vein is visualized by rotating the multi-plane dial to 65° at the same level or possibly 0.5 cm to 2 cm lower compared with the left upper pulmonary vein (see Fig. 4). (*B*) The close relationship between the superior vena cava and the right upper pulmonary vein is shown. This is an important relationship to consider when using PFO closure devices. This view is obtained using slight rotation from the bicaval view (see Fig. 1).

placed at roughly 30°. Visualization of the pulmonary veins, particularly the right upper pulmonary vein, is pertinent because the veins can become obstructed partially with improper positioning of the closure device.

Coronary sinus view

Obtaining a view of the coronary sinus can be difficult, especially to show the opening into the right atrium. The coronary sinus resides adjacent to the os of the inferior vena cava and more directly next to the tendon of Todaro (Fig. 6).

Mitral and tricuspid valves

Because the septal occluder device can impinge on the function of the mitral and tricuspid valves, it is important to obtain standard views, including orthogonal views of these valves as a baseline.

Evaluation of patent foramen ovale closure device

After the PFO closure device is in place, evaluation of optimal position is done by ICE (see later discussion). Long-term follow-up can be done by TEE or TTE. An example of a normally

positioned Cardioseal (NMT Medical, Inc., Boston, Massachusetts) PFO closure device is shown (Fig. 7A,B). A similar TEE view is shown (Fig. 7C) with an abnormally placed device. In this case, the left atrial side of the device has an arm that is protruding into the left atrium.

Pertinent views to obtain with the intracardiac echocardiography catheter

In this section, the echocardiographer (or interventional cardiologist who is performing the ICE examination) is taken through the views sequentially that are used during the implantation of the septal occluder device. For optimal orientation, we have combined the placement of the ICE catheter—as viewed by fluoroscopy—with the actual echocardiography image that is acquired. The reader should be cautioned that the position of the ICE catheter by fluoroscopy is meant to serve as a general guide. Obviously, each patient is different; therefore, the positions that we have shown for the ICE catheter will not always be successful.

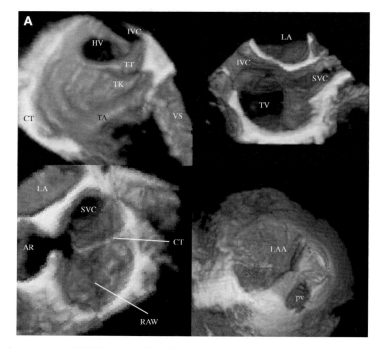

Fig. 6. Coronary sinus view by TEE shown in three-dimensional echo depicts the relationship between the coronary sinus, the inferior vena cava, the tricuspid annulus, and the tendon of Todaro. (TT-tendon of Todaro, TK-triangle of Koch, IVC-inferior vena cava, SVC, superior vena cava, CT-crista terminalis, TA-tricuspid annulus, RAW-right atrial wall, LAA-left atrial appendage, PV-pulmonary valve, AR-aortic root, VS-ventricular septum, HV-hepatic vein, TV-tricuspid annulus).

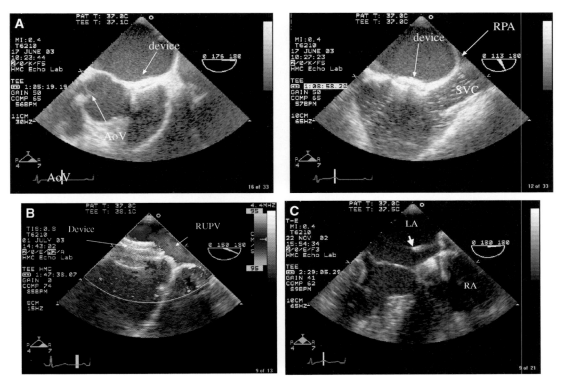

Fig. 7. (*A*) Example of a normally positioned PFO closure device by TEE. Note the symmetry of the arms on both the left and right side of the atria and the clear separation between the device and aortic valve (AoV). In the bicaval view, the device is seen adjacent to the right pulmonary artery (RPA) and superior vena cava (SVC). (*B*) Example of an Amplatz ASD occluder device that is appropriately positioned. In this case, the view shows the right upper pulmonary vein as well as well as the superior vena cava, Color Doppler shows no evidence of device leakage based on no color flow across the septum. (*C*) Example of a misaligned PFO device, in this case a (Cardioseal) device. In this case the left sided arm is protruding dramatically into the left atrium (arrow). This device also had substantial residual leak and surgical removal of the device and subsequent surgical repair of the patent foramen ovale was undertaken.

Basic atrial septal view

The basic atrial septal view (Fig. 8) is obtained with the ICE catheter placed at a 10 o'clock position relative to the spine using fluoroscopy as guidance. The position of the right heart can be inferred from the fluoroscopy view. This should provide a clear view of the interatrial septum and the left upper pulmonary vein.

Cephalad atrial septal view

With the catheter angled more cephalad, a more conventional view seen by TEE—the bicaval view—is appreciated. The difference is that the viewpoint is from the right atrium as opposed to the left atrium. Hence, the right atrium is on top and the left atrium is on the bottom, exactly the opposite from what cardiologists are used to seeing by TEE (Fig. 9).

Pulmonary vein view

Slight leftward (counterclockwise) rotation of the catheter will allow viewing of the left upper and left lower pulmonary veins. The right upper and right lower pulmonary veins are seen by further rightward (or clockwise) rotation of the ICE catheter (Fig. 10).

Coronary sinus view

With the ICE catheter in the standard view, movement of the catheter more inferior results in a view of the coronary sinus (Fig. 11). Evaluation of the position of the coronary sinus relative to

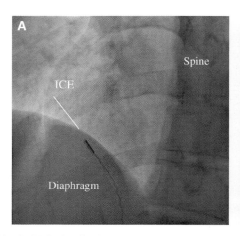
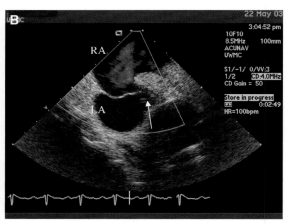

Fig. 8. PFO visualized by ICE catheter (*A*). With the ICE catheter, the (*B*) RA is at the top of the screen because the transducer is within the RA. The LA is on the bottom and the right-to-left flow through the PFO is depicted by the blue jet (*arrow*). Fluoroscopic view of the ICE catheter is shown for reference on the left. (Courtesy of Steven L. Goldberg, MD, Seattle, WA.)

the defect in the atrial septum is important so as to not damage or obstruct the coronary sinus.

Aortic valve view

The aortic valve view is useful, like the TEE view, to show the relationship of the defect relative to the aortic valve and aortic root (Fig. 12). A known complication of PFO occluder devices is erosion into the aorta. Hence, it is important to view these relationships and size the occluder device appropriately so that the device does not infringe on the aorta.

Atrial ventricular valve view

By positioning the ICE catheter across the PFO, the mitral valve can be viewed (Fig. 13). This particular view is pertinent before deployment of the device to estimate how close the atrial septal defect closure device will be to the AV valves.

Working view

The all-purpose working position of the ICE catheter is achieved with the catheter placed in the

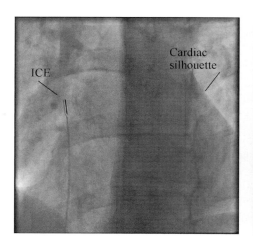
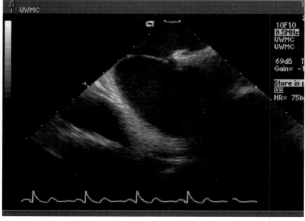

Fig. 9. With the ICE catheter placed more cephalad than in Fig. 7, the atrial septum is well visualized. (Courtesy of Steven L. Goldberg, MD, Seattle, WA.)

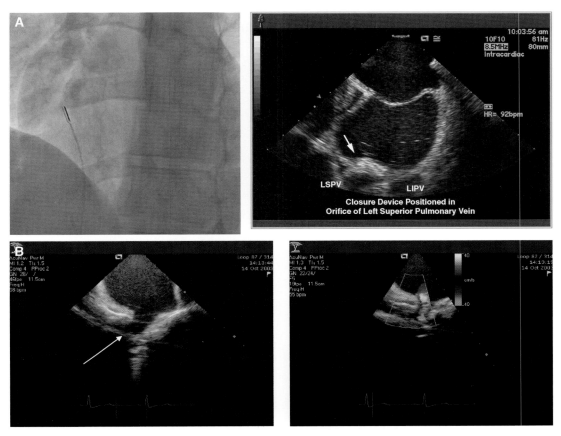

Fig. 10. (*A*) Pulmonary vein view by way of the ICE catheter. The occluder device is positioned in the left upper pulmonary vein (LSPV) in preparation for deployment. The left inferior pulmonary vein (LIPV) also is well visualized. (Courtesy of Siemens Medical Solutions, Inc., Malvern, PA.). (*B*) ICE of LIPV vein without color Doppler (*left*) and with color Doppler (*right*).

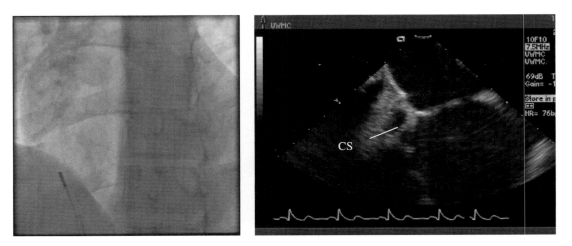

Fig. 11. Coronary sinus view. Note the coronary sinus (CS) at the inferior aspect of the interatrial septum. (Courtesy of Steven L. Goldberg, MD, Seattle, WA.)

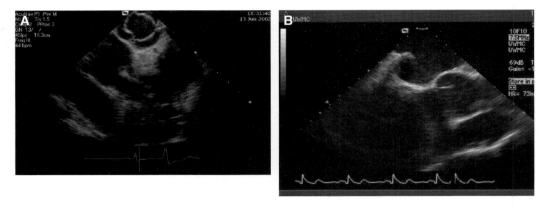

Fig. 12. Aortic valve view. The ICE catheter is moved to a more superior position than the working position to see the aortic valve. Shown are short axis view (*A*) and long axis view (*B*).

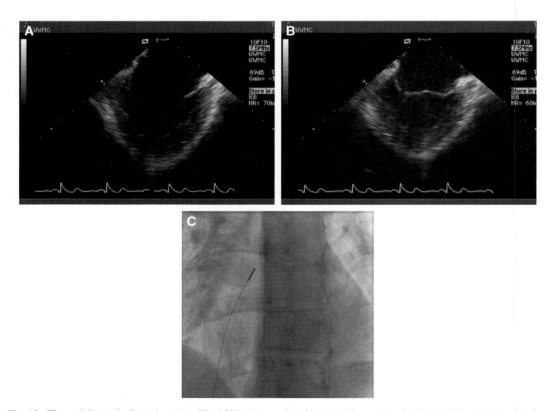

Fig. 13. The atrial ventricular valve view. The ICE catheter placed in a position across the interatrial septum and a view of the mitral valve. The valve is shown open in (*A*) and closed (*B*). The corresponding ICE catheter (*C*) position is shown in the fluoroscopy figure.

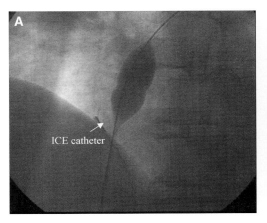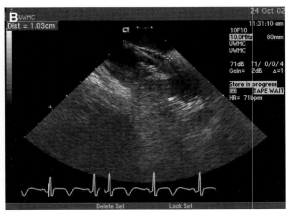

Fig. 14. A working view of the ICE catheter by fluoroscopy (*A*) and corresponding ICE images (*B*). In this stage of the procedure, a balloon is passed across the defect and inflated to determine the size of the defect. The size of the PFO is determined by measuring the waist of the balloon using electronic calipers by echocardiography. The size can be confirmed by measurement with fluoroscopy.

10 o'clock position to the spine with slight cephalad tilt. This allows a view of the interatrial septum, the superior vena cava, both atria, and the left upper pulmonary vein with just slight manipulation (see Fig. 8).

Sizing the defect

A catheter with a ballon on it is positioned with the balloon across the PFO. The balloon is inflated and the waste of the balloon is measured. This measurement of the waste is used to determine what size closure device will be deployed (Fig. 14).

Deployment of the device

With the ICE catheter still in working position, the occluder device—with a wire attached to it—is placed across the septum (Fig. 15). Position is confirmed by the ICE catheter. Some gentle push and pull maneuvers are applied to the device to be certain that it is stable and the wire is released.

Device deployed

The delivery cable has been removed and the device is in place and parallel to the septum, an optimal result. The left and right atria are seen

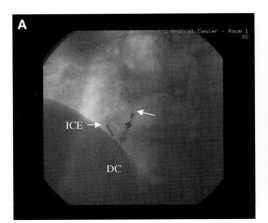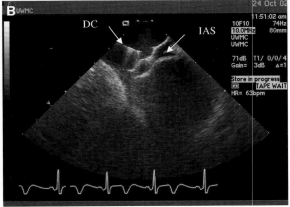

Fig. 15. (*A*) With the ICE catheter in the typical working position, the PFO closure device is seen in place across the interatrial septum with the deployment cable (DC) still attached to the device (*right arrow*). (*B*) The interatrial septum (IAS) is seen captured between the two sides of the closure device.

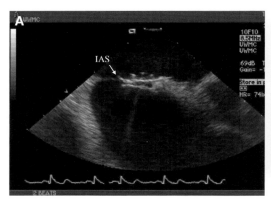

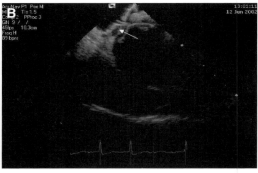

Fig. 16. (*A,B*) The closure device is now deployed with the delivery cable removed. The interatrial septum is seen captured between the two sides of the device.

well in Fig. 16A. In Fig. 16B, the left atrium is seen particularly prominently and the interatrial septum can be seen well-captured between the two sides of the occluder device.

Evaluation for interatrial septal leak by color Doppler

Color doppler interrogation of the interatrial septum at the level of the device shows no passage of color flow into the left atrium (Fig. 17). This is the optimal result and confirms no shunt.

Evaluation for interatrial septal leak by contrast (agitated saline)

Next, injection of agitated saline is performed to confirm that there is no intracardiac shunt (Fig. 18). In our experience, saline is more

sensitive and specific for picking up intracardiac shunting than is color Doppler. This is particularly true when the occluder device is in place because shadowing from the device is a significant problem.

Three-dimensional echocardiography

3D echocardiography by way of TEE is the other technology that is emerging as an adjunct in defining the size, shape, and number of atrial septal defects. Three-dimensional echocardiography has several advantages over two-dimensional (2D) echocardiography for the evaluation of an atrial septal defect. Some of these advantages can

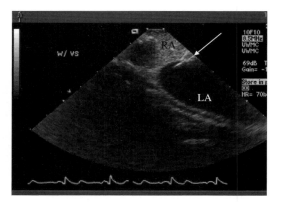

Fig. 18. Agitated saline contrast examination by ICE to evaluate for shunt. Note that contrast bubbles are seen only in the left atrium. This is indicative of the absence of intracardiac shunt. The arrow indicates the closure device.

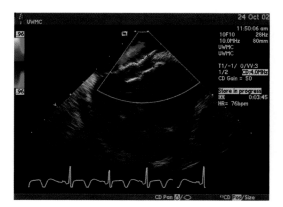

Fig. 17. Interrogation for leakage through the septal occluder device by color Doppler.

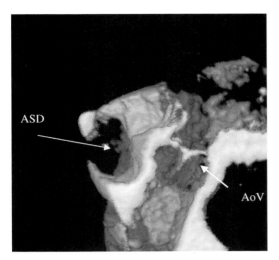

Fig. 19. Three-dimensional echocardiography view of an ASD shows the close relationship between this secundum and the aortic valve.

be applied to PFO. The advantages include: (1) a circumferential sizing of the defect, adding confidence to the maximum and minimal diameter as well as the true shape of the defect; (2) evaluation of the outer rim of the defect; (3) detection of fenestrations or multiple defects; and (4) simultaneous visualization of the surrounding structures in direct relationship to the ASD, particularly the pulmonary veins and vena cava. It is important to recognize that not all atrial septal defects are circular in shape. One

disadvantage of 3D echocardiography is that the inferior rim of a secundum ASD usually is not well-visualized because it is the furthest structure from the ultrasound transducer. In addition, 3D echocardiography that is performed by TEE is not real-time, but rather must be reconstructed from multiple 2D views. With specific regard to PFO, 3D echocardiography is definitely at a disadvantage because the typical PFO is extremely small (<3 mm in diameter). In addition, such defects typically open only with maneuvers (eg, Valsalva). Currently, the resolution of reconstructive 3D echocardiography is not adequate to see a PFO routinely. This is particularly challenging because the opening of a PFO is dynamic; this makes acquisition of multiple cardiac cycles that show a representative view of the PFO impossible. It is likely that this disadvantage will be overcome with real-time 3D imaging [4].

In addition, 3D echocardiography has advantages in the evaluation of the ASD closure device after it is deployed. The main advantage is simultaneous visualization of the surrounding structures that are in direct relationship with the ASD. The disadvantage is the reconstruction requirement; this makes 3D echocardiography largely impractical for immediate evaluation of the ASD closure device at the conclusion of the deployment. The good news is that this disadvantage will change soon with the advent of real-time 3D technology. Real-time 3D cardiography, currently marketed as "live 3D echocardiography" is available by way of TTE. Real-time 3D echo is not available in a transesophageal probe at this

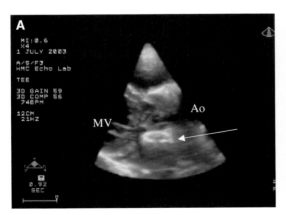

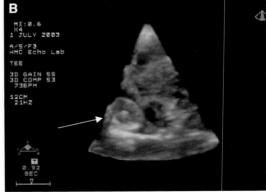

Fig. 20. This view of an Amplatz septal occluder device was obtained using live 3D echocardiography. Note the relationship of the aortic root to the Amplatz closure device. The device is on the superior edge of the left atrium. (A) The device is seen posterior to the aortic root and adjacent to the mitral valve in the left atrium. (B) The device is seen in the left atrium.

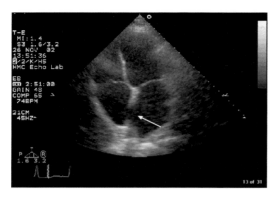

Fig. 21. An example of a transthoracic echocardiography showing dropout of the atrial septum. Because the atrial septum is in the far field, there can be lack of penetration of the ultrasound beam that leads to the appearance of an ASD. Many times, as in this case, there is no ASD. Color Doppler or contrast injection is required to evaluate for evidence of a shunt. The 2D images cannot be trusted always, especially in the case of transthoracic echocardiography. This type of problem rarely occurs with TEE.

time, but it likely will be within a few years. The advent of real-time 3D echocardiography using a transesophageal probe likely will add additional information about atrial septal problems that are not available with existing imaging modalities. It also is likely that the additional information will be of incremental value to the interventionalist who is closing septal defects.

Figure 19 shows and example of an atrial septal defect imaged by reconstructive 3D TEE. This image is produced using an ultrasound system with onboard 3D acquisition linked to the TEE probe (Philips Sonos 5500 and 7500; Philips Medical Systems, Andover, Massachusetts and Bothell, Washington). The 3D data set is acquired during the TEE examination and then reconstructed into the 3D image shown here using a computer workstation. The result is a particularly stunning appreciation of the relationships

between the interatrial septum and adjacent structures.

Live 3D views of an appropriately placed Amplatz (AGA Medical Corp., Golden Valley, Minnesota) septal occluder device for and atrial septal defect show in Fig. 20.

In Fig. 20, an example is shown of an Amplatz septal occluder device six months after placement. These images were obtained using transthoracic live 3D echocardiography (Philips 7500). The device is seen well-seated across the interatrial septum. The left atrial side of the device is seen in the images and once again the relationship with the aortic root is well-appreciated.

Summary

The use of TEE and ICE techniques have been extremely important in the development of closure of PFOs and ASDs using interventional techniques. These two imaging techniques have revolutionized the diagnosis and treatment of these problems and have gone far beyond TTE and its known problems for diagnosing septal defects (Fig. 21).

References

[1] Bjornstad PG. Transcatheter closure of atrial septal defects demands co-operation between the interventionist and the echocardiographer. Cardiol Young 2000;10(5):462–3.

[2] Cooke JC, Gelman JS, Harper RW, et al. Echocardiologists' role in the deployment of the Amplatzer atrial septal occluder device in adults. J Am Soc Echocardiogr 2001;14(6):588–94.

[3] Ren JF, Marchlinski FE, Callans DJ, et al. Clinical use of AcuNav diagnostic ultrasound catheter imaging during left heart radiofrequency ablation and transcatheter closure procedures. J Am Soc Echocardiogr 2002;15(10 Pt 2):1301–8.

[4] Downing SW, Herzog WR Jr, McElroy MC, et al. Feasibility of off-pump ASD closure using real-time 3-D echocardiography. Heart Surg Forum 2002; 5(2):96–9.

ELSEVIER
SAUNDERS

Cardiol Clin 23 (2005) 65–71

Hematologic Ramifications of Patent Foramen Ovale—role of Hypercoagulable State

Kathryn L. Hassell, MD

Department of Medicine, University of Colorado Health Sciences Center, 4200 East 9th Avenue,
C-222, Denver, CO 80262, USA

Closure of a patent foramen ovale (PFO) in patients with a history of cryptogenic stroke has been advocated and in the era of percutaneous closure is more easily and safely accomplished. This choice of treatment is directed by the premise that these patients experience paradoxical venous embolization, and closure could be expected to reduce significantly or eliminate the risk of recurrent stroke. Studies have demonstrated that both surgical and percutaneous closure of a PFO are associated with a reduced risk of recurrent stroke [1–9], although antiplatelet or anticoagulant therapy is sometimes continued after closure and may also affect stroke risk.

Because PFO is a relatively common anatomic abnormality, present in 20% to 25% of the general population, patients with PFO who experience a neurologic event probably have additional risk factors for thromboembolism. A hypercoagulable state, especially one that leads to an increased risk for venous thrombosis, might be expected to be prevalent in this population. Studies in this area have been limited, however.

Venous hypercoagulable states in patients with patent foramen ovale and neurologic events

Common and uncommon venous hypercoagulable states, along with their estimated prevalence in the general population, in control groups in case-control studies, and in patients with overt venous thromboembolic disease and with PFO, are listed in Table 1.

E-mail address: Kathryn.hassell@uchsc.edu

Testing for venous hypercoagulable states in patients with a PFO who have experienced a stroke or other apparent paradoxical embolism has been inconsistently performed. With the advent of percutaneous techniques, the number of patients evaluated for possible closure has increased. The majority of studies in the literature reporting results of percutaneous closure using various devices have excluded patients with possible causes of stroke other than the PFO. It is not clearly indicated, however, if patients with hypercoagulable states are excluded or which specific tests are performed to determine the presence of hypercoagulabilty [2,3,5,7]. In one series, testing was performed for levels of protein C, protein S, antithrombin, fibrinogen, and the presence of antiphospholipid antibodies, and activated protein C/factor V Leiden; if the findings were abnormal, the patients were deferred from closure. Details concerning the prevalence or types of hypercoagulability in the population screened were not provided [9]. Hypercoagulable states (types unspecified) were identified in 6% to 11% of patients who underwent percutaneous closure at two separate institutions [6,8]; an additional 11% had a history of venous thromboembolism [6]. In a single-institution study, testing was done for factor V Leiden, and unspecified assays were made for protein C, protein S, and antithrombin deficiencies, the presence of the lupus anticoagulant, anticardiolipin antibodies, and hyperhomocysteinemia [4]. Another small series of patients with cryptogenic stroke and PFO were evaluated for the presence of activated protein C resistance/factor V Leiden and anticardiolipin antibodies; other screening tests, if performed, were not mentioned [10]. The findings of these two reports

Table 1

Venous hypercoagulable states and their estimated prevalence in the general population/control groups, in patients with deep venous thrombosis and in patients with patent foramen ovale and neurologic events

Condition	Prevalence in general population or control groups (%)	Prevalence in patients with deep venous thrombosis (%)	Prevalence in patients with patent foramen ovale and stroke[a] (%)
Factor V Leiden	5–15 (white) <0.1 (nonwhite)	20–50	10
Prothrombin G20210A	2–5 (white) 0.012 (nonwhite other groups)	6–16	18
Elevated factor VIII	11	16–25	unknown
Hyperhomocysteinemia	unclear	5–33	0
Antiphospholipid antibodies (ACA, β_2GP-1 or LA)[++]	0–17	15–20	12
Lipoprotein(a)	0–7	20	unknown
Protein S deficiency	unclear	1–6	3
Protein C deficiency	0.2–0.4	3–4	0
Antithrombin deficiency	0.05–1	1–4	3
Dysfibrinogeremia	unknown	0.8	unknown

Abbreviations: ACA, anticardiolipin antibodies; β_2GP-1, anti-$\beta_2$glycoprotein-1 antibodies; LA, lupus anticoagulant.
[a] Based on small case series.

are summarized in Table 1. Case reports note the presence of hyperhomocysteinemia, protein S deficiency, and activated protein C resistance [11,12].

Although the available data are limited, the prevalence of venous hypercoagulable states seems to be somewhat underrepresented in patients with PFO and neurologic events, as compared with patients with more overt venous thromboembolic manifestations (see Table 1). If confirmed by larger studies, this lower prevalence may suggest that factors other than traditional venous hypercoagulable states may contribute to the risk of stroke in the PFO population. The apparent low incidence (4%) of associated deep venous thrombosis or pulmonary embolism at the time of ischemic

neurologic events may support this suggestion [13], although other sites of venous thrombosis, including the pelvic veins, are infrequently imaged in these patients.

Arterial hypercoagulable states in patients with patent foramen ovale and neurologic events

Testing for the presence of hypercoagulable states in patients who have experienced ischemic stroke or other neurologic events has varied, with limited testing often focusing on different subsets of patients. Hypercoagulable states associated with a risk for arterial thrombosis and their estimated prevalence in ischemic stroke populations are listed in Table 2. Factor V Leiden,

Table 2

Arterial hypercoagulable states and their estimated prevalence in the general population/control groups, in patients with stroke, and in patients with patent foramen ovale and neurologic events

Condition	Prevalence in general population/control groups (%)	Prevalence in ischemic stroke (%)		Prevalence in PFO/stroke population (%)[a]
		Population age ≤ 50	All ages	
Antiphospholipid antibodies (ACA, β_2GP-1, or LA)	0–17	2–45	2–34	3–43
Hyperchomocysteinemia	unclear	RR 1.3–1.5		0
Elevated lipoprotein (a)	0–7	33%		unknown
Dysfibrinogenemia	<12	<1%		unknown

Abbreviations: ACA, anticardiolipin antibodies; β_2GP-1, anti-$\beta_2$glycoprotein-1 antibodies; LA, lupus anticoagulant; PFO, patent foramen ovale; RR, relative risk.
[a] Based on small case series.

prothrombin G20210A, protein C, protein S, antithrombin, and Factor VIII are not listed on this table, because these hypercoagulable states are not consistently associated with an increased risk for arterial thrombosis [14–16].

Little information is available about the prevalence of arterial hypercoagulable states in patients with PFO and cryptogenic stroke. Table 2 gives the limited available data [4,10,12]. Assessment for the presence of antiphospholipid antibodies has been incomplete and often focuses on anticardiolipin antibodies. When assessment is limited in this way, the prevalence of antiphospholipid syndrome seems to be relatively low (3%–12.5%) [4,10]. When testing is expanded to include the lupus anticoagulant and anit-$\beta_2$glycoprotein-1 antibodies, however, a larger percentage of these patients (44%) seem to have antiphospholipid antibody syndrome [17]. This abstract noted the presence of arterial hypercoagulable states in 63% of patients with PFO and neurologic events. The presence of arterial hypercoagulable states may account for some the recurrent neurologic events that occur after closure, especially in patients with little or no residual leak.

Implications of hypercoagulable states for closure of patent foramen ovale

The goal of PFO closure in the patient with neurologic events is reduction of the risk of subsequent events by eliminating the route of presumed paradoxical embolism and eliminating the need for continued oral anticoagulation. Medical therapy for patients who have a PFO and a neurologic event has traditionally included long-term antiplatelet therapy or oral anticoagulation and is associated with a risk of recurrence of approximately 3% to 5% per year [18–20]. Patients with recurrent events who are receiving antiplatelet therapy may be switched to oral anticoagulation therapy. In general, transient ischemic events are more common than recurrent major stroke in patients receiving oral anticoagulation therapy [18]. This finding might be expected in patients with PFO and presumed paradoxical embolism, because antiplatelet therapy is relatively ineffective in preventing venous thrombosis. In theory, PFO closure would obviate the need for oral anticoagulant therapy.

Arterial hypercoagulable states

If a patient has an arterial hypercoagulable state, closure of the PFO may not significantly reduce the risk of recurrent stroke. In these cases, it may be impossible to determine if the patient's neurologic event resulted from a paradoxical embolism or from an intrinsic arterial thromboembolism associated with an underlying hypercoagulable state. The most common arterial hypercoagulable state, antiphospholipid antibody syndrome, can also cause venous thromboembolism and is usually treated indefinitely with oral anticoagulation therapy [21], whether or not the PFO is closed. Similarly, dysfibrinogenemias, although rare, would warrant indefinite oral anticoagulation therapy [22]. If the goal of PFO closure is to eliminate the need for oral anticoagulation therapy, closure may not be appropriate in patients with these or any other hypercoagulable states thought to confer a persistent risk for arterial thromboembolism.

Hyperhomocysteinemia is treated with vitamin therapy, commonly a combination of folic acid, vitamin B_6, or vitamin B_{12} [23]. Elevated lipoprotein(a) may be corrected by dietary modifications, niacin, or other lipid-lowering therapies [24]. Persistently elevated homocysteine or lipoprotein(a) levels in patients may cause continued arterial injury and represent an ongoing risk for recurrent stroke despite PFO closure.

Venous hypercoagulable states

It is not clear that the presence of venous hypercoagulable states should preclude PFO closure, because the mechanism of paradoxical embolism is eliminated by this approach. Chronic oral anticoagulation therapy would not be required for most patients with a venous hypercoagulable state once the PFO is closed, as long as there is no antecedent history of other, overt idiopathic venous thromboembolism [25]. There may, however, be a risk of procedure- or device-related thrombosis, as discussed later, which may warrant temporary initiation or continuation of oral anticoagulation therapy after PFO closure.

Procedure-related thrombosis

Because percutaneous closure involves catheterization of the deep venous system, there is theoretical concern about the development of periprocedural deep venous thrombosis in patients with a hypercoagulable state. The extent of this risk is unknown because studies of percutaneous closure either excluded patients with hypercoagulable states or did not assess patients for these states. There have been no published reports of periprocedural deep venous thrombosis in this patient population.

Device thrombosis

There have been several reports of device thrombosis after closure of atrial septal abnormalities. A series of 24 patients underwent percutaneous closure of an atrial septal defect or PFO using the ASDOS (Sulzer-Osypka, Germany) occlusion system, receiving periprocedural heparin followed by therapeutic oral anticoagulation therapy for 2 months [26]. Transesophageal echocardiography performed 3 days after implantation revealed a layer of echodense material assumed to be thrombus on both right and left atrial sides of the device in 20 of 22 patients; this layer receded over 1 to 6 months. Four patients developed additional, thicker, and in some cases mobile, areas of thrombus that resolved without symptoms of venous or arterial thromboembolism. Testing for protein C and protein S deficiencies, as well as for activated protein C resistance was performed and apparently was negative. Device thrombosis was noted in 2.9% of 276 patients who underwent placement of several generations of the PFO-Star device (Cardia, Burnsville, Minnesota) [9]. These thromboses were not associated with clinical symptoms, occurred with earlier-generation devices, and were not observed after clopidogrel was added to aspirin as postprocedural antiplatelet therapy. This study, however, excluded patients with recognized hypercoagulable states.

Case reports of device thrombosis [27,28], including the clamshell device [29] and Cardioseal (Nitinol Medical Technologies, Boston, Massachusetts) [30,31], note that the timing of thrombosis varies from several days to more than 1 year after device placement and is associated with recurrent neurologic events in these cases. Two patients required surgery for device explantation and pericardial patch [31], and thrombolytic therapy was used successfully to manage thrombosis for another patient [32]. Some type of screening for thrombophilias was usually performed, although the details are provided for only one patient, who was found to have factor V Leiden and was taking oral contraceptives at the time of her device thrombosis [31].

In other large case series reporting percutaneous closure of PFO using various devices [2,5–8], there are no reports of device thrombosis during 1 to 2 years of follow-up. In most of these studies,

postprocedural anticoagulation therapy was limited to low-dose aspirin therapy (81–100 mg) for up to 6 months. It is unclear how many, if any, hypercoagulable patients were included in these studies.

Given the potential complications of device thrombosis, including recurrent neurologic events, possible atrial arrhythmias, the need to resume anticoagulation therapy, or possible surgical removal of the device, it would seem prudent to consider relatively aggressive treatment in patients with hypercoagulable states, at least until endothelialization has taken place. The only case series to identify patients with recognized hypercoagulable states treated this subset of patients with postprocedural low molecular weight heparin until therapeutic oral anticoagulation with an international normalized ration (INR) of 2 to 3 was established [4]. This group of patients continued receiving oral anticoagulation therapy for at least 3 to 4 months or longer as dictated by their underlying hypercoagulable state. No device thromboses or bleeding complications were reported with a follow-up of just over 2 years.

Thus, although it is not clear that the presence of a venous hypercoagulable state should preclude PFO closure, given the presumed mechanism of paradoxical embolization, consideration of more aggressive postprocedural anticoagulation therapy may be warranted to prevent procedure-induced thrombotic complications.

Testing for hypercoagulable states

Testing for most hypercoagulable states can be performed in patients receiving stable oral anticoagulation or antiplatelet therapy, as delineated in Table 3 [25,33]. Protein C and protein S deficiencies are the only disorders that cannot be accurately assessed in patients being treated with oral anticoagulation therapy. Fortunately, these are relatively rare disorders, even in patients with overt venous thromboembolism, and it is unclear if oral anticoagulation therapy should be interrupted for the 2 to 3 weeks necessary to assess protein C and protein S levels accurately before device placement.

Evaluation for the presence of antiphospholipid antibody syndrome is fairly extensive. Testing should include measurement of anticardiolipin antibodies, anti-$\beta_2$glycoprotein-1 antibodies, and performance of at least two test methods for the lupus anticoagulant [21,34]. Diagnostic criteria

Table 3
Testing for hypercoagulable states

Condition	Test	Notes
Factor V Leiden	Activated protein C resistance assay	Does not discern hetero/homozygotes
	DNA analysis	Can be done at any time
Prothrombin G20210A mutation	DNA analysis	Can be done at any time
Elevated Factor VIII	Factor VIII activity	Measure more than once
		Increased risk if > 150%–200%
Antiphospholipid antibodies	dRVVT	Can be done in patients taking heparin,
	Other lupus anticoagulant tests	warfarin
	Anticardiolipin antibodies	Other tests include nonspecific inhibition,
	Anti-β_2-glycoprotein-1 antibodies	hexagonal array, and others
Hyperhomocysteinemia	Plasma homocysteine	Best measured fasting, repeat after
		supplementation
Elevated lipoprotein(a)	Lipoprotein (a) level	Increased risk > 30 mg/dL
Protein S deficiency	Protein S free antigen	Activity assays unreliable
		Lower in patients with vitamin K deficiency, liver disease, taking warfarin, with antiphospholipid antibodies
Protein C deficiency	Protein C activity	Lower in patients with vitamin K deficiency, liver disease, taking warfarin, with antiphospholipid antibodies
Antithrombin deficiency	Antithrombin activity	Lower in patients taking heparin or with liver disease
Dysfibrinogenemia	Euglobulin lysis time, thrombin time	Global fibrinolytic tests prolonged

include the presence of moderate to high titers of IgG or IgM anticardiolipin or anti-$\beta_2$glycoprotein-1 antibodies, or a lupus anticoagulant. If the first set of tests is positive, a second full set should be performed 6 to 8 weeks later to confirm the persistence of antiphospholipid antibodies. The diagnosis of antiphospholipid antibody syndrome is made when person who has had a thromboembolic event (arterial or venous) meets these laboratory diagnostic criteria; indefinite oral anticoagulation therapy is generally recommended [21,34].

Confirmatory testing on a second occasion is also recommended for elevated Factor VIII levels, protein C, protein S, and antithrombin deficiencies. Correction of hyperhomocysteinemia should be documented with repeat testing 3 to 4 weeks after initiation of vitamin supplementation.

Medical therapy in the absence of closure – a hematologist's perspective

The rate of recurrent neurologic events in patients with PFO treated with antiplatelet or oral anticoagulant therapy is reported to range from 2.4% to 5.5% [18–20]. In some of these reports more severe neurologic events seem to be more common in patients who are receiving antiplatelet therapy instead of oral anticoagulation therapy [18]. A recent large, randomized trial of unselected patients with ischemic stroke (the Warfarin-Aspirin Recurrent Stroke Study or WARRS) demonstrated that treatment with aspirin or warfarin resulted in the same rate of recurrent events [35]. The target INR range in that study was 1.4 to 2.8, and the average INR achieved was only 2.1. The relative benefits of current standard practice, with a target INR of 2 to 3, were not assessed by this study. In the Patent Foramen Ovale in Cryptogenic Stroke Study, a substudy of WARRS, the presence of PFO was not associated with an increased risk of recurrent events, and there was no difference between warfarin and aspirin therapy. Recurrence rates were quite high at 2 years (20.4% with aspirin and 16.6% with warfarin), however, and the mean INR in the warfarin group was only 2.0 [36]. The benefit of therapy with a higher target INR (2 to 3) was not assessed in this study. Thus, until the issue is specifically addressed in a randomized, controlled study, it seems reasonable to prescribe therapeutic oral anticoagulation therapy for patients with presumed paradoxical embolism, especially if a hypercoagulable state has been identified, unless PFO closure is performed.

Alternatively, antiplatelet therapy may be used initially; if recurrent events occur, oral anticoagulation therapy could be administered.

References

[1] Dearani J, Ugurlu B, Danielson G, et al. Surgical patent foramen ovale closure for prevention of paradoxical embolism–related cerebrovascular ischemic events. Circulation 1999;100(II):171–5.

[2] Du ZD, Cao QL, Joseph A, et al. Transcatheter closure of patent foramen ovale patients with paradoxical embolism: intermediate-term risk of recurrent neurological events. Catheter Cardiovasc Interv 2002;55:189–94.

[3] Butera G, Bini M, Chessa M, et al. Transcatheter closure of patent foramen ovale in patients with cryptogenic stroke. Ital Heart J 2001;2:115–8.

[4] Martin F, Sanchez P, Doherty E, et al. Percutaneous transcatheter closure of patent foramen ovale in patients with paradoxical embolism. Circulation 2002;106:1121–6.

[5] Windecker S, Wahl A, Chatterjee T, et al. Percutaneous closure of patent foramen ovale in patients with paradoxical embolism. Circulation 2000;101:893–8.

[6] Hung J, Landzberg M, Jenkins K, et al. Closure of patent foramen ovale for paradoxical emboli: intermediate-term risk of recurrent neurological events following transcatheter device placement. J Am Col Cardiol 2000;35(5):1311–6.

[7] Wahl A, Meier B, Haxel B, et al. Prognosis after percutaneous closure of patent foramen ovale for paradoxical embolism. Neurology 2001;57:1330–2.

[8] Bruch L, Parsi A, Grad MO, et al. Transcatheter closure of interatrial communications for secondary prevention of paradoxical embolism. Circulation 2002;105:2845–8.

[9] Braun M, Fassbender D, Schoen S, et al. Transcatheter closure of patent foramen ovale in patients with cerebral ischemia. J Am Col Cardiol 2002;39(12):2019–25.

[10] Chaturvedi S. Coagulation abnormalities in adults with cryptogenic stroke and patent foramen ovale. J Neurol Sci 1998;160:158–60.

[11] Cerrato P, Imperiale D, Bazzan M, et al. Inherited thrombophilic conditions, patent foramen ovale and juvenile ischaemic stroke. Cerebrovasc Dis 2001;11(2):140–1.

[12] Meier M, Landolt M. [Family anamnesis as the key to diagnosis. 1. Multi-infarct syndrome in atrial secundum type septal defect. 2. Thrombophilia of uncertain etiology: homocysteine in upper normal range]. Schweiz Rundsch Med Prax 2000;89(36):1442–3 [in German].

[13] Lamy C, Giannesini C, Zuber M, et al, for the Patent Foramen Ovale and Atrial Septal Aneurysm Study Group. Clinical and imaging findings in cryptogenic stroke patients with and without patent foramen ovale: The PFO-ASA study. 2002;33(3):706–11.

[14] Bushnell C, Goldstein L. Diagnostic testing for coagulopathies in patients with ischemic stroke. Stroke 2000;31:3067–78.

[15] Nabavi DG, Junker R, Wolff E, et al. Prevalence of factor V Leiden mutation in young adults and cerebral ischaemia: a case-control study on 225 patients. J Neurol 1998;245:653–8.

[16] Folsom A, Rosamond W, Shahar E, et al. Prospective study of markers of hemostatic function with risk of ischemic stroke. Circulation 1999;100(7):736–42.

[17] Dodge S, Hassell K, Keller J, et al. Arterial hypercoagulability is a common finding in patients referred for percutaneous device closure of patent foramen ovale for secondary prevention of systemic thromboembolization [abstract]. Presented at the American Heart Association 4th Scientific Forum on Quality of Care and Outcomes Research in Cardiovascular Disease and Stroke. November, 2002.

[18] Nedeltchev K, Arnold M, Wahl A, Sturzenegger M, et al. Outcome of patients with cryptogenic stroke and patent foramen ovale. J Interv Cardiol 2001;14(2):203–9.

[19] Mas JL, Zuber M. Recurrent cerebrovascular events in patients with patent foramen ovale, atrial septal aneurysm, or both and cryptogenic stroke or transient ischemic attack. French Study Group on Patent Foramen Ovale and Atrial Septal Aneurysm. Am Heart J 1995;130:1083–8.

[20] Bogousslavsky J, Garazi S, Jeanrenaud X, et al. Stroke recurrence in patients with patent foramen ovale: the Lausanne study. Lausanne stroke with paradoxic embolism study group. Neurology 1996;46:1301–5.

[21] Roubey R. Treatment of the antiphospholipid syndrome. Curr Opin Rheumatol 2002;14(3):238–42.

[22] Hayes T. Dysfibrinogenemia and thrombosis. Arch Pathol Lab Med 2002;126(11):1387–90.

[23] Key N, McGlennen RC. Hyperhomocyst(e)inemia and thrombophilia. Arch Pathol Lab Med 2002;126:1367–75.

[24] von Depka M, Nowak-Gottl U, Eisert R, et al. Increased lipoprotein(a) levels as an independent risk factor for venous thromboembolism. Blood 2000;96(10):3364–8.

[25] Bauer K. The thrombophilias: well-defined risk factors with uncertain therapeutic implications. Ann Intern Med 2001;135:367–73.

[26] Rosee KL, Deutsch HJ, Schnabel P, et al. Thrombus formation after transcatheter closure of atrial septal defect. Am J Cardiol 1999;84:356–9.

[27] Rodriquez CJ, Di Tullio MR, Sacco RL, et al. Intra-atrial thrombus after surgical closure of patent foramen ovale. J Am Soc Echocardiogr 2001;14(1):63–6.

[28] Gastmann O, Werner G, Babic U, et al. Thrombus formation on transcatheter ASD occluder device in a patient with coagulation factor XII deficiency. Cathet Cardiovasc Diagn 1998;43: 81–3.

[29] Stangl V, Stangl K, Bohn J, et al. Images in cardiothoracic surgery. Thrombus formation after catheter closure of an atrial septal defect with a clamshell. Ann Thorac Surg 2000;69(6):1956.

[30] Fabricius AM, Krueger M, Falk V, et al. Floating thrombus on an ASD occluder device in a patient with hemophilia A. Thorac Cardiovasc Surg 2001; 49(5):312–3.

[31] Nkomo V, Theuma P, Maniu C, et al. Patent foramen ovale transcatheter closure device thrombosis. Mayo Clin Proc 2001;76:1057–61.

[32] Vermeersch P. Thrombosis of a patent foramen ovale closure device: thrombolytic management. Catheter Cardiovasc Interv 2002;56:522–6.

[33] Greaves M. Thrombophilia. Clin Med 2001;1:432–5.

[34] Levine J, Branch W, Rauch J. The antiphospholipid syndrome. N Engl J Med 2002;346(10):752–63.

[35] Mohr JP, Thompson JL, Lazar RM, et al, for the Warfarin-Aspirin Recurrent Stroke Study Group A comparison of warfarin and aspirin for the prevention of recurrent ischemic stroke. N Engl J Med 2001;345(20):1444–51.

[36] Homma S, Sacco R, Di Tullio M, et al, for the PFO in Cryptogenic Stroke Study (PICSS) investigators Effect of medical treatment in stroke patients with patent foramen ovale. Circulation 2002;105: 2625–31.

Patent Foramen Ovale Closure: Historical Perspective

Samir R. Kapadia, MD

Department of Cardiovascular Medicine, Cleveland Clinic Foundation, 9500 Euclid Avenue,
F-25, Cleveland, OH 44195, USA

From the time when the only legal material for dissection was the bodies of hanged criminals, James Jeffray (Professor of Anatomy at Glasgow University from 1790 to 1848), in his classic monograph, supported the theory that in the fetus, blood crossed from the right atrium through the foramen ovale to the left atrium. Although the function of the foramen ovale was well-known, the first report of paradoxic embolization through a patent foramen ovale (PFO) has been attributed to Julius Cohnheim (1839–1884), a protégé of Virchow and Traube (Fig. 1). He described a fatal case of middle cerebral artery embolization in a 35-year-old woman who had deep venous thrombosis of the lower extremity. Since then, there have been many reports of a thrombus imaged while in transit from the right to left atrium through the PFO (Fig. 2) [1–3].

Repair of the interatrial septum was one of the first intracardiac defects to be tackled by surgery. Cohn, in 1947, first attempted experimental closure of an atrial septal defect (ASD) in dogs. The lateral right atrial wall was invaginated and stitched to the ASD margins. Using a tonsillar snare, the inverted atrial muscle was detached to form a patch to cover the defect. In 1948, Murray reported the first closure of an ASD in a 12-year-old child by an extracardiac method. A large suture was introduced to the right of the aorta and pulmonary artery, passed through the upper edge of the ventricular septum, and tied down between the superior vena cava and right pulmonary veins; this squeezed the entire interatrial septum. The first attempt to use the heart–lung machine was for a closure of an ASD by Dennis

and colleagues on April 5, 1951; however, the patient died of a massive air embolism. The first successful operation using the heart–lung machine, by Dr John Gibbon on May 6, 1953, also was to repair an ASD. Moreover, the first surface hypothermia with cessation of the circulation in Europe was performed for the direct suture of an ASD defect in Duesseldorf, Germany on February 9, 1955.

Similarly, because of the ease with which it can be approached, the atrial septum has long been an enticing target for catheter interventionalists. The first widely accepted interventional cardiac catheterization procedure was performed by William Rashkind, MD, who pioneered balloon atrial septostomy to enlarge ASDs in patients who had transposition of the great arteries [4]. In recent times, significant efforts have been made to achieve percutaneous closure of ASDs and the PFO.

The use of a device to close an ASD was first described by Hufnagel and Gillespie in an experimental model during surgery in 1951. They used two opposing buttons that were inserted through the atrial appendage and special rod introducers that were screwed together on opposite sides of the interatrial septum. Gross and his colleagues were the first to use a double-disc device to close ASDs in humans. One disc was placed in the left side of the septum and the other was placed on the right side; the two discs were buttoned together and anchored into the edges of the septum. This early strategy of surgical button occlusion was used in three humans; all of them died as a result of dislodgement of the double-disc prosthesis. Since then, surgical innovations, including endoscopic surgery, have been described for the closure of ASD; however, the fascination of a device to close a hole in the interatrial septum

E-mail address: skapadia@u.washington.edu

doi:10.1016/j.ccl.2004.10.012

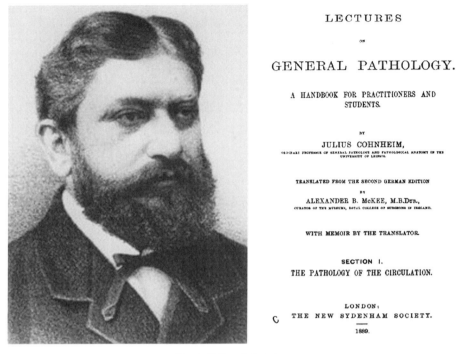

Fig. 1. Julius Cohnheim.

has remained with the interventional cardiology community.

Percutaneous devices

Percutaneous closure of an ASD was first performed in dogs, using an umbrella device, by King and Mills in 1973 (Fig. 3). The same investigators reported the first successful attempt at human percutaneous ASD closure in 1974 [5]. Their device consisted of two independent umbrellas—that consisted of six flat arms that radiated out from a central connection point; these had to be opened manually inside the atria and then snapped together. The King Mills occluder was implanted in several patients

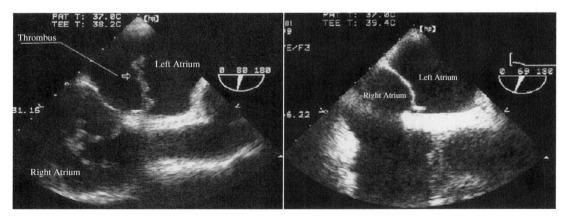

Fig. 2. (*Left*) Transesophageal echocardiographic (TEE) image showing thrombus in right atrium that extends into left atrium through PFO. (*Right*) In the same patient after heparin treatment, TEE image shows right and left atria with thrombus no longer seen. (*From* J Am Soc Echocardiogr 2002;15:1021; with permission.)

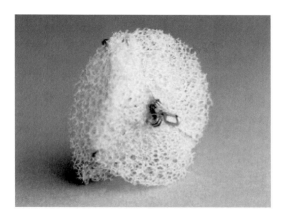

Fig. 3. Rashkind umbrella. (Courtesy of CR Bard, Murray Hill, New Jersey.)

successfully; however, the initial device was difficult to use because of multiple steps that were needed for deployment and a large (22F) delivery system [6]. These breakthrough procedures provided the proof of the concept that an atrial level shunt could be closed percutaneously with devices. This device was not developed further and never was available for routine clinical use.

Having witnessed this experience, Rashkind forged ahead with a second pioneering effort and shifted the focus to percutaneous closure of the patent ductus arteriosus. Using materials from the bioengineering laboratory at Children's Hospital of Philadelphia, he created a radial arm, single umbrella device with hooks at each end that could be collapsed and placed by way of a long sheath through the patent ductus. Demonstrating the principle in animal studies, human trials were performed in the late 1970s. Based on his relationship with the USCI Division of CR Bard (Murray Hill, North Carolina), from the septostomy program, USCI began product engineering efforts in conjunction with Rashkind to overcome some of the major design issues with the device, named the Rashkind patent ductus arteriosus (PDA) umbrella. Those efforts focused on trying to make the device stable in the ductus while eliminating the need for hooks, which frequently made the implant undeployable based on the patient's anatomy. Within 3 years, USCI, in conjunction with Rashkind and his colleague and close friend, Dr. Charles Mullins, had redesigned the implant. They made it significantly more "user friendly" by eliminating the barbs; creating a second, opposing umbrella disk; and modifying the technique to use the Mullins' transseptal sheath as a conduit for delivery. By the early 1980s, a multi-center clinical protocol was in place to close patent ductus. This implant, the Rashkind PDA umbrella, was, in essence, a "plug" that was designed to go in the ductus and was held in place by resistance of the arms rebounding against the ductal wall. This implant eventually received a US Food and Drug Administration (FDA) panel recommendation for approval, but never was brought to market in the United States.

Almost simultaneously, Rashkind continued his efforts on the closure by experimenting with a larger, single hexagonal disk device with six arms, three of which had barbed hooks at the ends to anchor the implant to the atrial septum. By 1985, this implant was in animal trials in Philadelphia under Dr. Rashkind's supervision. This implant also was designed for delivery through a 16 F transseptal length sheath. The physician team that helped to develop this implant included Dr. James Lock of Children's Hospital Boston, Dr. William Hellenbrand of Yale University Medical Center, Dr. Larry Latson of the University of Nebraska, and Dr. Lee Benson of the Hospital for Sick Children, Toronto. The delivery system for this implant was the same as the PDA umbrella and consistently got tangled in the ASD device. Therefore, a new attachment system—the pin system (developed by Rudy Davis at USCI)—was incorporated into the delivery catheter for ASD and PDA. This new system prevented entanglement of the delivery catheter into the implant during release and paved the way for human clinical trials. This attachment mechanism is still in use today.

The first human use of the Rashkind ASD umbrella implant occurred under an investigational device exemption (IDE) pilot study at Yale University in early 1987. The case was a complete success; six patients were implanted with the device at Yale University or Children's Hospital of Omaha. It became clear that the defect needed to be precisely in the center of the septum, because although the implant had an ingenious method for helping to center the implant, any error or misalignment meant that a hooked arm could get caught on a pulmonary vein orifice or other aspect of the left atrium. Davis remembers the first two patients who were operated on at Yale University well for two reasons. First, because none of Dr. Hellenbrand's colleagues in attendance would scrub in with him, the duty was left to Davis. Second, Dr. Mullins had an acute myocardial infarction only a few days after his return to

Houston which required multiple bypass grafts. From this moment on, Dr. Mullins became even more dedicated to the principle of transcatheter closure and vowed to do all he could to keep children from the "barbarism of surgery."

Subsequent to these procedures, on his return to Boston, Dr. Lock, in a personal communication with Davis, indicated that "this device is a great proof of principle but will only work in a small percentage of perfectly centered ASDs. It's too dangerous otherwise." Lock rededicated his efforts away from the PDA, believing that between coils and the Rashkind PDA umbrella this technical challenge mostly was solved. He refocused his efforts on the ASD, defining the ideal implant as one that is as effective as surgical closure, safe, simple to use, with little metal mass, and that promotes a healthy healing response. Ultimately, Lock described the need for an implant that eventually would be resorbed by the body, leaving only a new, vascularized, fully intact septum behind [7].

What resulted was a collaborative effort in Boston to find a better design. Lock, who by now had accumulated a significant experience with the PDA occluder, postulated that something of this nature that was readily retrievable might work in an ASD. In the fall of 1987, Davis and Lock conceived and drew the first designs for the clamshell umbrella (this design was drawn on a napkin over hot dogs and beer during a Boston Red Sox baseball game). This implant significantly changed the configuration of the PDA implant by: (1) adding multiple spring coils at the center, (2) placing a center (elbow) spring coil along each arm so that greater springback and improved septal conformability was achieved, (3) positioning the disks such that there would be a patch on the septum, and (4) creating sizes that could be used in larger defects. Within 6 months, prototypes were created and animal trials were completed. The first human patients were implanted in the fall of 1988 at Children's Hospital Boston. The initial clamshell worked well (one of the first patients was a mountain climber who returned to the hills less than 1 week after implant, unheard of at the time), but was believed to be more unstable than desired (despite no embolizations); a decision was made to make the wire framework diameter 30% larger. In experienced hands, the clamshell device offered an elegant, but simple, implant that could be deployed under fluoroscopic guidance alone [8].

The basic functioning and deployment of the device was similar to that seen with most of the devices that are used today for ASD or PFO closure. The two opposing, self-expanding umbrellas of the device clamped the atrial septal remnant between them. The device was delivered through a long sheath that was positioned in the left atrium. The distal umbrella was advanced out the end of the sheath and was allowed to expand. The entire system was withdrawn slightly so that the arms of the distal umbrella contacted the atrial septum. After proper positioning of the distal umbrella was ensured and the proximal umbrella was determined to be on the right side of the septum, the sheath was withdrawn further to uncover the proximal umbrella in the right atrium.

The advantages of the clamshell were that it did not depend on hooks to anchor and it could be recaptured or removed at various steps of delivery if the positioning of the device was not satisfactory. This device was used in almost 900 patients in the early 1990s with reasonable safety; and it was within the USCI run clinical study that patients who had ASD, ventricular septal defect (VSD), Fontan fenestration, and the first PFO related stroke were treated. The first 36 patients who had PFO related stroke who were treated were reported on by Bridges et al in 1992 [9]. The device had to be withdrawn from clinical trials in 1991 because of frequent (up to 84%) fracture of one or more metal arms of the umbrellas within the first year after device implantation (Fig. 4). The fractures were not associated clearly with any adverse clinical events and almost all of these patients are doing well with their implants [10]. The investigation into the cause of the arm fracture revealed that the stainless steel that was used in the device was brittle enough to fracture routinely when subjected to mild flexion forces in the beating heart. Furthermore, the manufacturing techniques that was used at that time created stresses in areas of the implant that made it more susceptible to fracture propagation. The device was re-engineered significantly using a nonferrous metal, state of the art metallurgy (MP35n), and manufacturing techniques, and is now available as the CardioSEAL (NMT Medical, Boston, Massachusetts) device.

CardioSEAL and Amplatzer (AGA Medical Corp., Golden Valley, Minnesota) PFO closure devices are approved for PFO closure by the FDA under the Humanitarian Device Exemption. The Amplatzer ASD closure device was approved by the FDA for use for the secundum ASD closure. CardioSEAL also is premarket approval approved for ventricular septal defects. Other

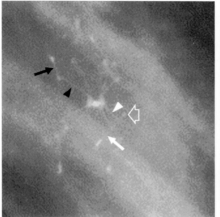 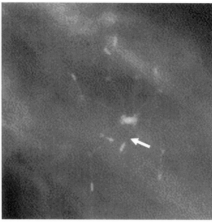

Fig. 4. Fractured struts. (*Left*) Magnified lateral chest radiograph showing fractured inferior right atrial arm 2 months after device placement. Normally, each arm has a proximal portion (*black arrowhead*) that is attached by a hinge to a distal portion (*black arrow*) with a radiodense tip. The distal portion of the fractured arm (*white arrow*) is displaced slightly from the fracture point at the hinge (*open arrow*), whereas the proximal portion (*white arrowhead*) remains in place. (*Right*) Same patient 3 months after fracture. The distal portion (*white arrow*) of the fractured arm is seen closer to the center of the device. (*From* Prieto LR, Foreman CK, et al. Intermediate-term outcome of transcatheter secundum atrial septal defect closure using Bard Clamshell Septal Umbrella. Am J Cardiol 1996;78(11):1311; with permission.)

devices are in clinical trials, including the Buttoned Device (Custom Medical Devices, Amarillo, Texas) the Helex Device (W.L. Gore, Flagstaff, Arizona), the PFO Star (Cardia, Burnsville, Minnesota), and the STARFlex Occluder (NMT Medical). Several other attempts at device design (ASDOS Device, Osypka Corp., Berlin, Germany; Angel Wings Device; Monodisk Device) were tested in clinical trials during the early to mid 1990s and have not been pursued commercially in the United States. All of these devices were designed for ASD closure but it probably is logical to use them for PFO closure also, with the exception of the Amplatzer ASD device; this would result routinely in significant residual leaks. There is now a specific Amplatzer PFO device. Each of these devices is summarized briefly in the following paragraphs.

The CardioSEAL septal occluder

The clamshell device was significantly re-engineered to prevent arm fractures, improve complete closure rates, and improve ease of use. It now is known as the CardioSEAL device (Fig. 5). Compared with the original device, three major changes were made; different material was used for the arms (alloy MP35n), two elbow joints were

used on the longer arms to improve flexibility and reduction in metal fatigue, and state of the art manufacturing methods were developed. This device received FDA approval for PFO closure under humanitarian use guidelines in February of 2000. The use of this device requires monitoring by the institutional review board. It is approved for use in patients who have recurrent cryptogenic stroke that is due to presumed paradoxic embolism through a PFO and who have failed conventional drug therapy [11].

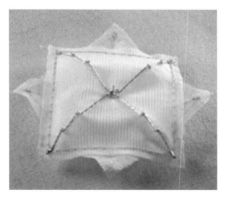

Fig. 5. The CardioSEAL device. (Courtesy of NMT Medical, Boston, MA.)

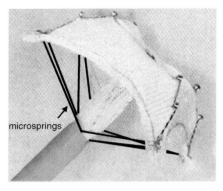

Fig. 6. The STARFlex device. (Courtesy of NMT Medical, Boston, MA.)

The STARFlex septal occluder

The STARFlex implant is an updated version of the CardioSEAL implant [12]. It is structurally identical to the CardioSEAL implant, with the addition of a self-centering mechanism that is made of nitinol springs that are connected between the two umbrellas and a flexible core wire with a pin-pivoting connection (Fig. 6). This device was designed primarily for ASD closure but quickly was adopted for PFO closure as a result of improved clinical performance compared with the original CardioSEAL. It is used widely in Europe, primarily as a PFO closure device [13]. Although it is unknown if the design changes in the STARFlex implant will reduce the number of device arm fractures, Horst Seivert, MD reported at the 2002 American Heart Association meeting that in his nearly 100 patients who had a STAR-Flex implanted for PFO, he has had only one device arm fracture with no sequelae. STARFlex

should allow for more complete closure of ASDs and PFOs. In the United States, the CLOSURE I study has been launched. This clinical trial is a prospective, multi-center, randomized controlled trial to evaluate the safety and efficacy of the STARFlex septal closure system versus best medical therapy in patients with a stroke and/or transient ischemic attack (TIA) due to presumed paradoxical embolism through a PFO.

Amplatzer atrial septal defect occluder

The Amplatzer line of occluders started with the development of the Amplatzer ASD Occluder in the mid-1990s. Kurt Amplatz, MD, an interventional radiologist who consulted for ev3 (Plymouth, Minnesota), created the first implant in the product line and formed his own company, AGA Medical. The ASD implant was released in Europe in 1997 after having undergone sufficient clinical trials to support a conformite Europenne mark application [14]. Early in the ASD experience, attempts were made to close PFOs in patients who had experienced strokes. Because of marginal success, the ASD device was modified and a separate PFO occluder was developed [15]. AGA Medical went on to develop specific VSD and PDA devices.

The Amplatzer ASD septal occluder, as are all of the AGA devices, is a self-expandable, double-disc device that is made from shape memory dense nitinol wire mesh (Fig. 7). The two discs are linked together by a short connecting "stent" or waist that corresponds to the size of the ASD. To increase its closing ability, the discs and the waist are filled with polyester fabric. The polyester fabric is sewn securely to each disc by a polyester thread. The

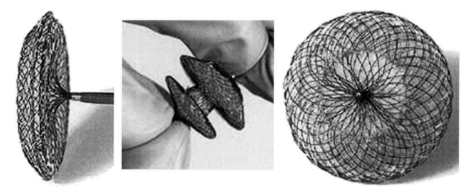

Fig. 7. The Amplatzer device. (Courtesy of AGA Medical, Golden Valley, MN.)

Amplatzer ASD device received FDA approval for ASD closure in December of 2001. It is the predominant ASD closure device in the United States and Europe, with product sizes up to 38 mm. The AGA ASD Occluder has a significant clinical history and generally provides excellent results in an ASD. Of the known ASD closure devices, it is the only one that is fully retrievable and reusable before release; this unique feature results from the nitinol wire mesh design. Atrial erosion with severe pericardial effusion has been reported. Care must be taken with AGA devices to ensure an adequate rim surrounding the defect being treated because the rigidity and metal mass of the device are the most significant of any of the devices.

Buttoned device

Button devices date to the late 1980s, when Terry Sideris, MD invented the first version that was designed to close the patent ductus arteriosus. In 1990, Sideris et al [16] described the animal work with a device that they called the "Buttoned" device. This device is composed of a square sheet of polyurethane foam that is supported by two independent, diagonally-situated wire arms (the occluder) and a separate counter occluder. The regular buttoned device consists of a square-shaped occluder that is implanted onto the left atrial side of the atrial septum and a rhomboid-shaped counter-occluder that is placed on the right atrial side. This device has the least inherent rigidity and strength, which can be an advantage or a disadvantage in various situations. The foam occluder can be folded easily into the delivery catheter by compressing the sides of the square so that the support wires are parallel to each other, rather than in an "X" configuration. The foam resumes its square shape when advanced out of the delivery catheter in the left atrium and remains attached centrally to a nylon thread that is looped through a hollow loading wire that extends out of the end of the delivery catheter. Control of the occluder is maintained by this flexible connection. However, after the occluder has been advanced out of the delivery catheter, it only can be removed from the body with difficulty and may be distorted if removal is attempted. If the occluder is the proper size and has been deployed correctly in the left atrium, it is pulled against the left side of the atrial septum. The counteroccluder is advanced over the loading wire and buttoned onto a knotted loop that is attached

to the center of the occluder. The counteroccluder wire and the higher left atrial pressure prevent the occluder from migrating into the left atrium. The device is released by cutting one side of the nylon thread loop and pulling the thread out of the loading wire. Because of instances of unbuttoning (7.2% in the international study) and subsequent embolization of the counteroccluder and of instances of migration of the core of a support wire, several modifications were made in the device [17]. The fourth generation device has two spring buttons—instead of the single button in the earlier devices—to prevent "unbuttoning" (Fig. 8). The modified fourth generation device with a centering mechanism—"centering-on-demand buttoned device"—also has been described to allow reduction in size without adversely affecting dislodgement or occlusion rates.

For PFO closure, modification of this device—"inverted button device"—has been described. In the inverted buttoned device, the counteroccluder and occluder are reversed. The counteroccluder is made up of rhomboid-shaped, 1/16-inch polyurethane foam that is mounted on a single, Teflon-coated wire skeleton to be placed into the left atrium. The occluder is made up of an X-shaped Teflon-coated wire skeleton that is covered with 1/16-inch thick polyurethane foam that is placed in the right atrium [18]. The Buttoned device is available in the United States as an experimental device in an ongoing multi-institutional trial; however, it is more widely accessible in other countries.

Angel Wings device

In 1993, Das et al [19] at the University of Minnesota, reported the results using the device, now known as the Angel Wings device (Microvena Inc.), in 20 dogs. This device consists of two square nitinol wire frames; each supports a square of stretchy Dacron fabric that is sewn to the perimeters. The device is deployed through a sheath that initially is placed in the left atrium. A control handle is used to advance the distal square out of the sheath slowly. The device is not designed to be removed easily after the distal square has expanded. The entire system is pulled back until the distal square is against the atrial septum. The control handle is used to advance the proximal disc as gentle traction is maintained on the delivery catheter. The proximal square resumes its expanded shape in the right atrium and the conjoint ring that connects the two

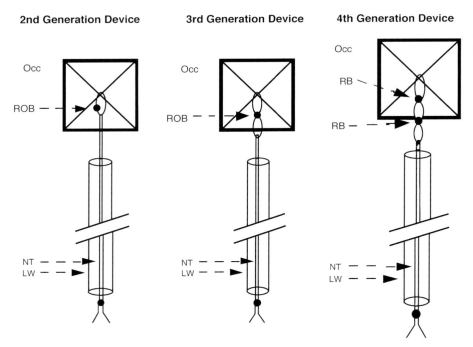

Fig. 8. The occluder component of the second, third, and fourth generation buttoned device. The occluder (Occ) in all devices is composed of an X-shaped wire skeleton that is covered with 1/16-inch polyurethane foam. In the second generation device (*left*), a 2-mm string loop is attached to the center of the occluder. The loop is closed with a knot (button) that is made radiopaque. This radiopaque button (ROB) can be visualized easily by fluoroscopy. In the first generation device (not shown), the button was not radiopaque. A folded 0.008-inch nylon thread (NT) passes through the hollow loading wire (LW) after passing through the loop in the center of the occluder. In the third generation device (*middle*), an extra loop is added immediately beneath the ROB. This modification converted the eccentric button of the second generation device to be aligned straight, thus making it easier to button the Occ and counteroccluder across the atrial septum. In the fourth generation device (*right*), the button loop is replaced with two "spring" radiopaque buttons (RB) that are mounted 4 mm apart. The intent was to reduce unbuttoning that was seen with earlier generation devices. (*From* Rao PS, Chandar JS, Sideris EB. Role of inverted buttoned device in transcatheter occlusion of atrial septal defects or patent foramen ovale with right-to-left shunting associated with previously operated complex congenital cardiac anomalies. J Am Coll Cardiol 2000;36:584; with permission.)

square results in a degree of self-centering of the device within the ASD. A release fixture remains attached to one corner of the right atrial square until the operator decides whether the device is positioned appropriately. Angel Wings was used in clinical trials in the United States for more than two years and was commercially available in Europe for a short period of time in 1997–1998 [20]. The Angel Wings device is no longer used clinically in the United States or Europe; it was discontinued because of problems with atrial perforations. A new generation of device, "Guardian Angel," reportedly is nearing availability in the United States under FDA protocol.

Transcatheter patch occlusion

All of the above described devices are double-disc devices with wire components. Therefore, they are subject to limitations and complications that are associated with such designs. The use of transcatheter polyurethane patches in the occlusion of atrial defects was designed to improve on device-related problems (Fig. 9). Transcatheter-delivered patches also are useful in occluding defects that cannot be closed with conventional double-disc devices; however, there is limited clinical experience with these devices [21,22]. Results of larger international clinical trials and FDA-approved (with IDE) human trials are awaited.

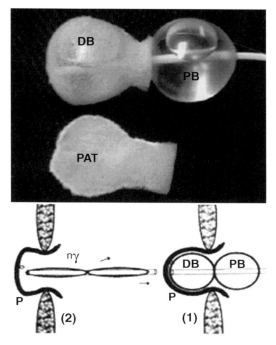

Fig. 9. (*Top panel*) Sleeve patch. The patch can be seen before (*below*) and after mounting on the distal balloon of the double balloon catheter. Proximal balloon (PB) and distal balloon (DB) are inflated. PB: proximal balloon; pat/P: patch. (*Bottom panel*) Diagram of a double-balloon sleeve patch occlusion (1) and patch release (2). Occlusion involved inflation of the distal balloon/patch in the left atrium first, opposite the defect, and inflation of the proximal balloon. Release involved deflation of the distal and proximal balloons, removal of the balloon catheter, and release of the patch after pulling the double nylon thread as a single strand. (Sideris EB, Sideris CE, Stamatelopoulos SF, et al. Transcatheter patch occlusion of experimental atrial septal defects. Catheter Cardiovasc Interv 2002;57:405; with permission; and Sideris EB, Toumanides S, Macuil B, et al. Transcatheter patch correction of secundum atrial septal defects. Am J Cardiol 2002;89(9):1083; with permission.)

Helex device

The Helex occluder is composed of a single piece of nitinol wire with a patch of microporous expanded polytetrafluoroethylene (ePTFE; W.L. Gore & Associates, Inc) attached along its length (Fig. 10). The nitinol wire frame consists of two equal-sized opposing disks that bridge and occlude the septal defect. The occluder is fixed in place by a unique locking mechanism that passes through the center of the device from the left to the right atrial disk. The ePTFE is designed to

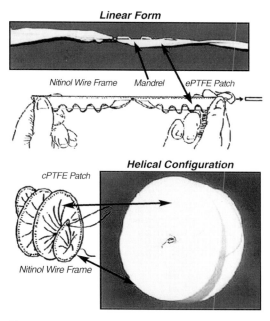

Fig. 10. Helex septal occluder shown in linear (*upper panel*) and helical (*lower panel*) configurations. A single piece of ePTFE is attached throughout its length to a nitinol frame wire; this leaves little metal exposed to bloodstream. Note mandrel that courses through center of device before implantation in upper panel. (Zahn EM, Wilson N, Cutright W, et al. Development and testing of the Helex septal occluder, a new expanded polytetrafluoroethylene atrial septal defect occlusion system. Circulation 2001;7;104(6):712; with permission.)

facilitate rapid cell penetration—thereby promoting rapid tissue ingrowth—and result in permanent defect closure and device stability. Before the device is locked in place, repeated repositioning of either disk or complete device removal by way of the delivery catheter is possible [23]. Information from large human trials is awaited.

Atrial septal defect occlusion system

In 1991, Babic et al [18] described a device with two separate umbrellas that are made of nitinol wire and covered with polyurethane. It was designed to be delivered over a guidewire loop that extends from the femoral vein, through the ASD, and out of the femoral artery (Atrial septal defect occlusion system; Osypka Corporation) [24]. Each umbrella is composed of five arms of preshaped nitinol wire that are covered by a thin polyurethane patch (Fig. 11). A venous sheath is advanced over the guidewire to the left atrium.

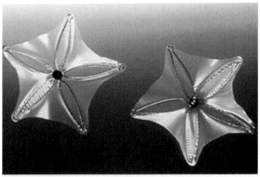

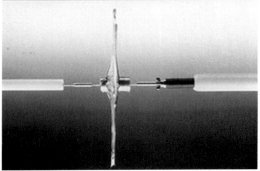

Fig. 11. (*Upper panel*) Two umbrella-shaped patches that are positioned on either side of the defect. (*Lower panel*) Installed halves are screwed together after positioning by way of two catheters and a guidewire.

The distal umbrella is advanced to the left atrium through this sheath; a conus on the guidewire prevents the umbrella from advancing further. The umbrella self-expands and is pulled back against the left atrial side of the septum by pulling on the venous side of the guidewire rail. The proximal umbrella is advanced through the sheath and is allowed to expand in the right atrium. Each umbrella is delivered separately to each side of the atrial septum after a wire is passed from the femoral vein to the femoral artery through the defect. The umbrellas are screwed together across the ASD. Although this complex device has been used successfully in clinical trials, it may find only limited use in clinical practice and is not available in the United States [25].

Summary

The work of the pioneers in PFO closure finally may evolve into a front-line therapy for secondary prevention of stroke in selected patients who have PFO and embolic events. Current implants, although new to most of interventional cardiology and neurology, are the result of years of steady, progressive work. It seems that PFO closure is here to stay and will become a key element in a collaborative approach between cardiology and neurology in the treatment of embolic stroke. The advances in device technology may make PFO closure sufficiently safe, effective, and durable that it may become one of the most frequent catheter laboratory procedures to be performed.

Acknowledgments

I am sincerely indebted to Mr. Rudy Davis (VP, Clinical Development NMT Medical, Inc.) for providing invaluable and interesting information on the development of the closure devices.

References

[1] Aggarwal K, Jayam VK, Meyer MA, et al. Thrombus-in-transit and paradoxical embolism. J Am Soc Echocardiogr 2002;15:1021–2.

[2] Falk V, Walther T, Krankenberg H, et al. Trapped thrombus in a patent foramen ovale. Thorac Cardiovasc Surg 1997;45:90–2.

[3] Claver E, Larrousse E, Bernal E, et al. Giant thrombus trapped in foramen ovale with pulmonary embolus and stroke. J Am Soc Echocardiogr 2004;17: 916–8.

[4] Rashkind WJ, Miller WW. Creation of an atrial septal defect without thoracotomy. A palliative approach to complete transposition of the great arteries. JAMA 1966;196:991–2.

[5] King TD, Mills NL. Nonoperative closure of atrial septal defects. Surgery 1974;75:383–8.

[6] King TD, Thompson SL, Steiner C, et al. Secundum atrial septal defect. Nonoperative closure during cardiac catheterization. JAMA 1976;235:2506–9.

[7] Lock JE, Rome JJ, Davis R, et al. Transcatheter closure of atrial septal defects. Experimental studies. Circulation 1989;79:1091–9.

[8] Meier B, Lock JE. Contemporary management of patent foramen ovale. Circulation 2003;107:5–9.

[9] Bridges ND, Hellenbrand W, Latson L, et al. Transcatheter closure of patent foramen ovale after presumed paradoxical embolism. Circulation 1992;86: 1902–8.

[10] Martin F, Sanchez PL, Doherty E, et al. Percutaneous transcatheter closure of patent foramen ovale in patients with paradoxical embolism. Circulation 2002;106:1121–6.

[11] NMT Medical. FDA Disclaimer. Available at: http://www.nmtmedical.com/products/ci/fda_dislcaimer.htm. Accessed December 8, 2004.

[12] Hausdorf G, Kaulitz R, Paul T, et al. Transcatheter closure of atrial septal defect with a new flexible, self-centering device (the STARFlex Occluder). Am J Cardiol 1999;84:1113–6.

[13] Carminati M, Chessa M, Butera G, et al. Transcatheter closure of atrial septal defects with the STAR-Flex device: early results and follow-up. J Interv Cardiol 2001;14:319–24.

[14] Sharafuddin MJ, Gu X, Titus JL, et al. Transvenous closure of secundum atrial septal defects: preliminary results with a new self-expanding nitinol prosthesis in a swine model. Circulation 1997;95:2162–8.

[15] Han YM, Gu X, Titus JL, et al. New self-expanding patent foramen ovale occlusion device. Catheter Cardiovasc Interv 1999;47:370–6.

[16] Sideris EB, Sideris SE, Fowlkes JP, et al. Transvenous atrial septal defect occlusion in piglets with a "buttoned" double-disk device. Circulation 1990;81:312–8.

[17] Rao PS, Berger F, Rey C, et al. Results of transvenous occlusion of secundum atrial septal defects with the fourth generation buttoned device: comparison with first, second and third generation devices. International Buttoned Device Trial Group. J Am Coll Cardiol 2000;36:583–92.

[18] Rao PS, Chandar JS, Sideris EB. Role of inverted buttoned device in transcatheter occlusion of atrial septal defects or patent foramen ovale with right-to-left shunting associated with previously operated complex congenital cardiac anomalies. Am J Cardiol 1997;80:914–21.

[19] Das GS, Voss G, Jarvis G, et al. Experimental atrial septal defect closure with a new, transcatheter, self-centering device. Circulation 1993;88:1754–64.

[20] Das GS, Harrison JK, O'Laughlin MP. The Angel Wings Das devices for atrial septal defect closure. Curr Interv Cardiol Rep 2000;2:78–85.

[21] Sideris EB, Sideris CE, Stamatelopoulos SF, et al. Transcatheter patch occlusion of experimental atrial septal defects. Catheter Cardiovasc Interv 2002;57:404–7.

[22] Sideris EB, Toumanides S, Macuil B, et al. Transcatheter patch correction of secundum atrial septal defects. Am J Cardiol 2002;89:1082–6.

[23] Zahn EM, Wilson N, Cutright W, et al. Development and testing of the Helex septal occluder, a new expanded polytetrafluoroethylene atrial septal defect occlusion system. Circulation 2001;104:711–6.

[24] Babic UU, Grujicic S, Popovic Z, et al. Double-umbrella device for transvenous closure of patent ductus arteriosus and atrial septal defect: first experience. J Interv Cardiol 1991;4:283–94.

[25] Sievert H, Babic UU, Hausdorf G, et al. Transcatheter closure of atrial septal defect and patent foramen ovale with ASDOS device (a multi-institutional European trial). Am J Cardiol 1998;82:1405–13.

ELSEVIER
SAUNDERS

Cardiol Clin 23 (2005) 85–89

CARDIOLOGY
CLINICS

Patent Foramen Ovale and the Platypnea-Orthodeoxia Syndrome

Grace Pei-Wen Chen, MD[a], Steven L. Goldberg, MD[a],
Edward A. Gill, Jr, MD[a,b,*]

[a]Division of Cardiology, Department of Medicine, University of Washington School of Medicine,
1959 Pacific Avenue NE, Seattle, WA 98195, USA
[b]Harborview Medical Center, 325 Ninth Avenue, Seattle, WA 98104, USA

Orthopnea is a relatively frequent complaint encountered in clinical practice. Congestive heart failure is a classic example of a condition characterized by orthopnea. In contrast, platypnea is much less common and therefore is less understood. The word "platypnea" refers to dyspnea induced by an upright posture and relieved by recumbence. A finding on physical examination that corroborates this complaint is orthodeoxia, namely, arterial oxygen desaturation that is incurred by an upright posture and improved by a recumbent one. Platypnea and orthodeoxia are often associated, and the term "platypnea-orthodeoxia" is frequently used to describe the syndrome of abnormal oxygenation in the upright position. Several clinical entities have been associated with the platypnea-orthodeoxia syndrome, and these entities can involve a variety of organ systems (Box 1).

The precise underlying mechanisms by which these clinical entities produce platypnea and orthodeoxia are unknown. Nevertheless, several mechanisms have been postulated. They fall into three main categories: intracardiac shunting, pulmonary vascular shunting, and ventilation-perfusion mismatching. The first category involves intracardiac shunting, which is the main focus of this article. The presence of a right-to-left heart shunt is of course an important differential diagnosis to consider in cases of dyspnea and deoxygenation. Patients with symptomatic right-to-left heart shunts are usually dyspneic regardless of posture, however. Some intracardiac shunts are anatomically small and clinically silent. Most patients with these small shunts are asymptomatic and do not come to medical attention. In select instances, these small intracardiac shunts are physically stretched by an upright posture, allowing more shunting through the defect and producing clinical symptoms and signs. This sequence of events is postulated to be the mechanism by which intracardiac shunting through a patent foramen ovale [1], an atrial septal defect [2], or an atrial septal aneurysm [3] can cause platypnea and orthodeoxia.

In addition to the anatomic size of the intracardiac shunts, one must consider the physiologic driving force for shunting. Again, a small amount of shunting usually does not produce symptoms. Symptomatic arterial deoxygenation occurs only with a significant amount of blood flow from the right to the left heart through these intracardiac communications. Under most physiologic conditions, the left atrial pressures are higher than the right atrial pressures, and blood shunts from the left to the right side. This kind of shunting has its own set of clinical consequences, but it does not produce arterial deoxygenation. Significant right-to-left heart shunting takes place primarily when there is concomitant pulmonary hypertension. The elevated right-sided pressures provide the driving force for deoxygenated blood to flow from the right heart to the left

* Corresponding author. Division of Cardiology, Department of Medicine, University of Washington School of Medicine, 1959 Pacific Avenue NE, Box 359748, Seattle, WA 98195.
E-mail address: eagill@u.washington.edu (E.A. Gill).

Box 1. Clinical entities associated with platypnea-orthodeoxia

Cardiac
Patent foramen ovale
Atrial septal defect
Atrial septal aneurysm
Pericardial diffusion
Dilated aorta
Persistent Eustachian valve
Constrictive pericarditis

Pulmonary
Emphysema
Arteriovenous malformations
Pneumonectomy
Pulmonary embolism

Gastrointestinal
Hepatopulmonary syndrome

Musculoskeletal
Deficient abdominal musculature
Kyphoscoliosis

Neural
Autonomic dysfunction

heart through the intracardiac communications. An otherwise clinically silent patent foramen ovale, for example, can manifest with the platypnea-orthodeoxia syndrome during an attack of pulmonary embolism [4]. When searching for the cause of platypnea-orthodeoxia, it therefore behooves the clinician to seek not only the presence of an intracardiac communication but also a possible concomitant pulmonary pathology.

Sometimes right-to-left heart shunting occurs even though the pulmonary pressures are normal. In these special cases the intrathoracic anatomy and physiology allow blood to flow from the right atrium to the left atrium against a higher left atrial pressure. For instance, an extrinsic compression of the right atrium (eg, with hydrothorax after pneumonectomy [5]) can increase right heart pressures and facilitate right-to-left shunting without affecting pulmonary pressures. Similarly, a decrease in right ventricular compliance can facilitate right-to-left heart shunting despite normal pulmonary pressures. This decreased right ventricular compliance is the postulated mechanism by which platypnea-orthodeoxia develops in cases of right ventricular ischemia or pneumonectomy [6–8].

In constrictive pericarditis, the dependence on high right-sided filling pressure to maintain an adequate right-sided cardiac output may cause platypnea-orthodeoxia because right heart preload decreases in the upright position [9].

Most importantly, changes in the anatomic relationship between the vena cava and the atrial septum can cause preferential blood flow from the vena cava through the interatrial defect despite normal pulmonary pressures. A persistent Eustachian valve can help direct blood flow from the vena cava to the interatrial communication [10]. A loculated pericardial effusion [11] or a dilated aortic root [12] can alter the atrial anatomy and cause platypnea-orthodeoxia. Kyphoscoliosis or prior thoracotomy (including pneumonectomy) [13] has also been reported to cause to platypnea and orthodeoxia. In these cases, it is thought that the anatomic alteration facilitates shunting through the interatrial communication, leading to arterial deoxygenation.

Not all cases of platypnea-orthodeoxia have a single obvious cause. Often, in fact, several potential mechanisms combined lead to the syndrome. One such case involves a 79-year-old woman whose kyphotic posture and dilated thoracic aorta altered the intrathoracic relationships and might have allowed more shunting across the patent foramen in the upright position [14]. Another case involves a 71-year-old man with a severe right-to-left shunt through a patent foramen ovale in the absence of elevated right-sided pressures [15]. The authors hypothesized that the opening of the foramen ovale was the result of mechanical deformation of the atrial septum by both his thoracic aortic aneurysm and an atrial septal aneurysm. A third case involves an 80-year-old woman with an elongated, ectatic thoracic aorta pressing on the right atrium, creating a deformity in the atrial septum that might have caused the foramen ovale to open when she was in the erect position [16]. A new thoracic spine compression fracture might have further altered her thoracic anatomy, facilitating the shunt.

Noncardiac mechanisms of platypnea-orthodeoxia are related mainly to pulmonary vascular shunting and ventilation-perfusion mismatching. First, arterial desaturation occurs when deoxygenated blood passes through pulmonary vascular shunts without receiving oxygen. If there is a greater concentration of shunting in the lower lung fields, an upright posture can lead to more severe arterial desaturation because gravity pulls a greater amount of blood flow through these shunts. A classic example of pulmonary vascular shunting is an arteriovenous malformation, which has been implicated in case reports of platypnea-orthodeoxia [17]. Second, postural changes in regional pulmonary perfusion can exacerbate ventilation-perfusion mismatching, causing platypnea-orthodeoxia. The capillaries in the alveolar walls are distended by the hydrostatic pressures from within and compressed by the alveolar pressures from without. Alveolar pressures are uniformly distributed throughout the normal lung, but in an upright person perfusion pressure is lowest at the apex and highest at the lung base. Under different normal and pathologic conditions, one may find any one of three possible zones of pulmonary blood flow [18]. Zone one is characterized by a lack of blood flow because alveolar pressures exceed perfusion pressures. Zone two is characterized by intermittent blood flow because systolic arterial pressure exceeds alveolar pressure but diastolic pressure falls below alveolar pressure. Zone three is characterized by continuous blood flow because perfusion pressures exceed alveolar pressures at all times. In a normal person, the apical lung regions have more zone-one physiology, resulting in a moderate degree of dead space ventilation. At the bases, there is more zone-three physiology, resulting in shunting. In both extremes of the lung, inequalities of ventilation and perfusion decrease the effectiveness of the lung for gas exchange. Ventilation-perfusion mismatching can be exaggerated in certain conditions, leading to significant postural changes in arterial oxygenation. In some patients with chronic obstructive pulmonary disease, for example, the parenchymal destruction causes significant physiologic dead space and shunts; the accentuated ventilation-perfusion mismatching can occasionally manifest with the platypnea-orthodeoxia syndrome [19].

Pulmonary perfusion abnormalities are sometimes seen in patients with liver disease. The hepatopulmonary syndrome is the triad of liver disease, an increased alveolar-arterial gradient when breathing room air, and evidence of intrapulmonary vascular dilatation [20]. Clinical findings are predominated by symptoms and signs of liver disease, but the most striking features of the syndrome are clubbing and platypnea-orthodeoxia. Autopsy specimens from patients with the hepatopulmonary syndrome have documented the existence of precapillary pulmonary vascular dilatations and direct arteriovenous communications [21,22]. Pulmonary arteriovenous communications have been discussed previously. In vascular dilatations, oxygen molecules may be unable to diffuse to the center of the dilated vessel to provide adequate oxygenation. Because the vascular abnormalities seem to predominate in the lower lung fields, patients can experience worsening hypoxemia when moving from the supine to the upright posture. The hepatopulmonary syndrome is a major differential to keep in mind during a work-up for platypnea-orthodeoxia, because subtle changes on the echocardiogram may sway the diagnosis from intracardiac shunts to intrapulmonary shunts, as discussed later.

Normally the autonomic nervous system helps maintain vascular tone and minimize postural changes in perfusion and thereby minimize ventilation-perfusion mismatching. When patients with autonomic dysfunction assume an upright posture, they can experience a drop in perfusion pressure and greater zone-one physiology, leading to ventilation-perfusion mismatching. Moreover, patients with autonomic neuropathy may have an attenuated hypoxic vasoconstrictor response. These patients may have persistent blood flow through poorly oxygenated areas of lung, leading to pulmonary shunting and arterial desaturation. There have been several case reports of platypnea-orthodeoxia attributable to autonomic dysfunction [23,24]. Finally, effective ventilation requires intact functioning of the respiratory mechanics. A rare cause of platypnea-orthodeoxia is deficient abdominal musculature, which results in loss of diaphragmatic support in the upright posture as the abdomen protrudes anteriorly. During recumbence, the abdominal viscera resume support of the diaphragm, stretching it to its optimal operational length. This form of platypnea-orthodeoxia syndrome can be alleviated with the use of abdominal binders [25].

Although the platypnea-orthodeoxia syndrome is thought to be rare, many affected patients may not be diagnosed correctly from routine ECG and chest roentgenogram. A high index of suspicion is necessary, and attention must be paid to the pattern of the occurrence of the dyspnea. If the syndrome is suspected, measurement of arterial blood gases in supine and upright positions should be made to document orthodeoxia. In addition to making this measurement on room air, one should also perform the measurement with inhalation of 100% oxygen to aid detection of intrapulmonary or intracardiac shunting. As explained earlier, pulmonary and cardiac pathologies are the main causes of platypnea-orthodeoxia, and the diagnostic work-up should focus on these areas. The work-up for pulmonary pathologies is not detailed in this article. Intracardiac shunting can be investigated by several modalities. With transcranial Doppler, an intracardiac shunt can be diagnosed by detection of air microemboli in a middle cerebral artery after peripheral injection of agitated saline. Quantification of the shunt is possible by right heart catheterization with arterial sampling. The preferred diagnostic modality, however, is echocardiography. Echocardiography allows one to visualize the atrial and ventricular septum for defects, aneurysms, or other abnormalities. Peripherally injected agitated saline may be used to detect small right-to-left heart shunts. The Valsalva maneuver may enhance detection of a right-to-left shunt, but the acoustic window may be lost during the maneuver. Transesophageal echocardiography has greater spatial resolution than transthoracic echocardiography in diagnosing interatrial shunts and is considered the reference standard for the diagnoses of patent foramen ovale [26]. Transesophageal echocardiography can also detect other shunts, such as a sinus venosus defect, that may be difficult to see on transthoracic echocardiography [27]. Combining transesophageal echocardiography with contrast injection allows characterization of the motion of the septum in relation to the timing of the passage of saline contrast [28]. Finally, the effects of postural changes on intracardiac structure and blood flow are not easily seen with diagnostic modalities such as cardiac catheterization, and a significant shunt inducing platypnea-orthodeoxia may not be appreciated. Tilt-table contrast echocardiography, on the other hand, is an elegant method for detecting a significant orthostatic increase in the degree of right-to-left shunt [4,27,29].

Several points should be borne in mind when working up potential cardiac causes of platypnea-orthodeoxia. First, as discussed earlier, concomitant pulmonary pathology must be ruled out. Second, multiple cardiac conditions sometimes combine to produce the syndrome. Third, it may be challenging to differentiate intrapulmonary from intracardiac shunting, because contrast crosses from the right to the left heart in both conditions. This issue is especially important when suspicion for intrapulmonary shunting is relatively high, for example in cirrhotic patients. In general, the appearance of contrast crossover within four cardiac cycles of right atrial opacification argues in favor of intracardiac shunting, whereas late crossover (after more than four cardiac cycles) suggests intrapulmonary shunting.

Once an intracardiac shunt is identified as the culprit for platypnea-orthodeoxia, surgical or percutaneous closure of the shunt can be considered. There have not been randomized studies on the efficacy of surgical or percutaneous closure in patients with the platypnea-orthodeoxia syndrome from intracardiac communications. Anecdotal reports suggest symptomatic relief and an improved quality of life [2,3,5,13,16,27,29], but this finding may be subject to reporting bias. Some conditions, such as pulmonary embolism inducing a significant flow across the interatrial defects, are transient; after resolution of the precipitating event, the patient may no longer exhibit any symptoms that require closure of the defect. Other conditions, such as postpneumonectomy, are more permanent facilitators of shunting; if the patient is severely symptomatic, definitive closure of the interatrial defect may be necessary [4]. As experience with catheter-based treatment increases, more and more patients with the platypnea-orthodeoxia syndrome are being referred for closure of their patent foramen ovale. Adverse events are not trivial and have been documented with every occluder [30]. The decision to intervene therefore rests heavily on the severity of symptoms and on concerns for other morbidities associated with the defects (eg, embolic stroke).

Summary

The platypnea-orthodeoxia syndrome is a rare but important condition caused by a variety of clinical entities. Several mechanisms have been postulated to cause platypnea and orthodeoxia. These mechanisms mainly involve intracardiac shunting, pulmonary vascular shunting, and ventilation-perfusion mismatching. Patent foramen ovale is an important type of intracardiac shunt that can produce platypnea-orthodeoxia in select patients. Concomitant pulmonary hypertension must be ruled out, but symptoms can occur without pulmonary hypertension in cases with altered intrathoracic anatomy and physiology. Diagnosis usually entails transthoracic or transesophageal echocardiogram, ideally with postural provocation by the tilt-table test. Treatment with surgical or percutaneous closure may result in symptomatic relief. The decision to intervene is based mainly on the severity of symptoms and potential morbidities associated with the defect.

References

[1] Sorrentino M, Resnekov L. Patent foramen ovale associated with platypnea and orthodeoxia. Chest 1991;100(4):1157–8.

[2] Hirai N, Fukunaga T, Kawano H, et al. Platypnea-orthodeoxia syndrome with atrial septal defect. Circ J 2003;67:172–5.

[3] Acharya SS, Kartan R. A case of orthodeoxia caused by an atrial septal aneurysm. Chest 2000; 118(3):871–4.

[4] Seward JB, Hayes DL, Smith HC, et al. Platypnea-orthodeoxia: clinical profile, diagnostic workup, management, and report of seven cases. Mayo Clin Proc 1984;59:221–31.

[5] Begin R. Platypnea after pneumonectomy. N Engl J Med 1975;293:342–3.

[6] Strunk BL, Cheitlin MD, Stulbarg MS, et al. Right-to-left interatrial shunting through a patent foramen ovale despite normal intracardiac pressure. Am J Cardiol 1987;60:413–5.

[7] Dlabal PW, Stutts BS, Jenkins DW, et al. Cyanosis following right pneumonectomy: importance of patent foramen ovale. Chest 1982;81:370–2.

[8] Smeenk FWJW, Twisk SPM, Berreklouw E, et al. Dyspnea after pneumonectomy. Eur Respir J 1991; 4:243–5.

[9] Mashman WE, Silverman ME. Platypnea related to constrictive pericarditis. Chest 1994;105:636–7.

[10] Bashour T, Kabbani S, Saalouke M, et al. Persistent Eustachian valve causing severe cyanosis in atrial septal defect with normal right heart pressures. Angiology 1983;34:79–83.

[11] Adolph EA, Lacy WO, Hermoni YI, et al. Reversible orthodeoxia and platypnea due to right-to-left intracardiac shunting related to pericardial effusion. Ann Intern Med 1992;116:138–9.

[12] Medina A, de Lezo JS, Caballero E, et al. Platypnea-orthodeoxia due to aortic elongation. Circulation 2001;104(6):741.

[13] Landzberg M, Sloss LJ, Faherty CE, et al. Orthodeoxia-platypnea due to intracardiac shunting: relief with transcatheter double umbrella closure. Cathet Cardiovasc Diagn 1995;36:247–50.

[14] Varkul M, Robinson T, Ng E, et al. Orthodeoxia and platypnea secondary to a patent foramen ovale despite normal right-sided cardiac pressures. Can Respir J 2001;8(2):105–7.

[15] Faller M, Kessler R, Chaouat A, et al. Platypnea-orthodeoxia syndrome related to an aortic aneurysm combined with an aneurysm of the atrial septum. Chest 2000;118(2):553–7.

[16] Popp G, Melek H, Garnett AR Jr. Platypnea-orthodeoxia related to aortic elongation. Chest 1997;112(6):1682–4.

[17] Robin ED, Laman D, Horn BR, et al. Platypnea related to orthodeoxia caused by true vascular lung shunts. N Engl J Med 1976;294:941–3.

[18] Guyton, Hall. Textbook of medical physiology. W.B. Saunders.

[19] Michel O, Sergysels R, Ham H. Platypnea induced by worsening of VA/Q inhomogeneity in the sitting position in chronic obstructive lung disease. Chest 1988;93(5):1108–10.

[20] Krowka MJ, Cortese DA. Hepatopulmonary syndrome current concepts in diagnostic and therapeutic considerations. Chest 1994;105:1528–37.

[21] Berthelot P, Walker JG, Sherlock S, et al. Arterial changes in the lungs in cirrhosis of the liver – lung spider nevi. N Engl J Med 1966;274:291–8.

[22] Schraufnagel DE, Kay JM. Structural and pathologic changes in the lung vasculature in chronic liver disease. Clin Chest Med 1996;17(1):1–12.

[23] Fox JL, Brown E, Harrison JK, et al. Platypnea-orthodeoxia and progressive autonomic failure. Am Rev Respir Dis 1989;140:1802–4.

[24] Ferry TG, Naum CC. Orthodeoxia-platypnea due to diabetic autonomic neuropathy. Diabetes Care 1999;22(5):857–9.

[25] Fauci AS, et al. Harrison's principles of internal medicine. McGraw-Hill.

[26] Kerut EK, Norfleet WT, Plotnick GD, et al. Patent foramen ovale: a review of associated conditions and the impact of physiological size. J Am Coll Cardiol 2001;38:613–23.

[27] Roxas-Timonera M, Larracas C, Gersony D, et al. Patent foramen ovale presenting as platypnea-orthodeoxia: diagnosis by transesophageal echocardiography. J Am Soc Echocardiogr 2001;14(10): 1039–41.

[28] Langholz D, Louie EK, Konstadt SN, et al. Transesophageal echocardiographic demonstration of distinct mechanisms for right to left shunting across a patent foramen ovale in the absence of pulmonary hypertension. J Am Coll Cardiol 1991;18:1112–7.

[29] Herregods MC, Timmermans C, Frans E, et al. Diagnostic value of transesophageal echocardiography in platypnea. J Am Soc Echocardiogr 1993; 6:624–7.

[30] Landzberg MJ, Khairy P. Indications for the closure of patent foramen ovale. Heart 2004;90:219–24.

ELSEVIER
SAUNDERS

Cardiol Clin 23 (2005) 91–96

CARDIOLOGY
CLINICS

Patent Foramen Ovale: Does it Play a role in the Pathophysiology of Migraine Headache?

Rachel Donahue Beda, MD[a], Edward A. Gill, Jr, MD[a,b],*

[a]Division of Cardiology, Department of Medicine, University of Washington School of Medicine,
1959 Pacific Avenue NE, Seattle, WA 98195, USA
[b]Harborview Medical Center, 325 Ninth Avenue, Seattle, WA 98104, USA

Migraine headache is a common and disabling condition. Recent statistics from the World Health Organization list migraine headache nineteenth among diseases causing worldwide morbidity [1]. Migraine headaches affect all races, although not equally, affecting whites more than other races and females more than males. Most estimates put the prevalence of migraine headache at 10% to 12% in the general population, but actual rates vary. A large-scale survey of the Baltimore County, Maryland, population, for example, found that for whites, migraine headaches were present in 20.4% of females and 8.6% of males; African-Americans were affected at rates of 16.2% of females and 7.2% of males, and Asians were affected at rates of 9.2% of females and 4.2% of males [2]. The suffering associated with migraine headaches accounts for significant lost productivity in missed hours of work and for significant costs in health care dollars spent. In one 1992 report, migraine headaches were estimated to cost between $5.6 and $17.2 billion in sick days and lost productivity, depending on the prevalence of migraine headache [3]. Another HMO-based study found that patients with migraine headache submit up to twice as many health care claims and up to 2.5 times as many pharmacy claims as nonsufferers [4].

Migraine headache is commonly divided into two major subtypes: migraine headache with aura, or classic migraine headache, and migraine headache without aura, or common migraine headache. For all the studies examined in this article, the diagnosis of migraine headache was based on criteria standardized by the International Headache Society [5]. Migraine headache without aura is the most prevalent subtype, accounting for as many as 80% of migraine headache attacks. Several studies have shown migraine headache to be a risk factor for ischemic stroke, especially in young women [6,7]. This risk, combined with the higher incidence of patent foramen ovale (PFO) in the population of younger stroke patients [8] has led to the speculation that PFO could play a causative role in the pathogenesis of migraine headache. PFO has a natural prevalence of approximately 25% in the general population [9]. Because the prevalence of migraine headache in the general population is less than 25%, there is clearly not a one-to-one correlation between the presence of PFO and development of migraine headache, but, as discussed in the following sections, PFO is significantly more frequent in the population of migraine headache sufferers than in the general population.

Prevalence of patent foramen ovale among migraine headache patients

Several studies to date have examined the prevalence of PFO among patients with migraine headache, both with and without aura (Table 1). Most of these studies are relatively modest in size, with one larger study encompassing 581 patients. The first study to address the relationship between PFO and migraine headache specifically was Del Sette et al [10] in 1998, which was a case-control

* Corresponding author. Division of Cardiology, Department of Medicine, University of Washington School of Medicine, 1959 Pacific Avenue NE, Box 359748, Seattle, WA 98195.

E-mail address: eagill@u.washington.edu (E.A. Gill).

Table 1
Prevalence of patent foramen ovale among migraine headache patients versus controls

Study	Total # of patients	Migraine patients with PFO (%)	Controls with PFO (%)	Odds ratio	95% confidence interval	P
Del Sette et al, 1998	94	18/44 (41%)	8/50 (16%)	3.2	1.4–7.2	<0.005
Anzola et al, 1999	191	With aura 54/113 (48%)	5/25 (20%)	3.66	1.21–13.25	0.01
		Without aura 12/53 (23%)		1.17	0.32–4.45	NS

study of 44 patients with migraine headaches with aura, 77 patients under the age of 50 years with focal cerebral ischemia, and 50 case controls. Transcranial Doppler was used to assess for appearance of microbubbles in the cerebral vasculature after injection of agitated saline into the antecubital vein, both during normal respiration and immediately following Valsalva maneuver. The appearance of three or more microbubbles within 15 seconds of injection qualified as a positive study for intracardiac shunt. Eighteen of 44 migraine headache patients (41%) had evidence of right-to-left intracardiac shunting, as did 26 of 73 of the focal cerebral ischemia patients (35%). In contrast, only 8 of 50 of the case controls (16%) had evidence of right-to-left shunting, significantly different than the rate observed in the migraine headache patients (relative risk, 3.2; 95% confidence interval [CI], 1.4–7.2; $P < 0.005$).

Anzola et al [11] performed a case-control study of 113 patients suffering from migraine headache with aura, 53 patients who had migraine headache without aura, and 25 age-matched controls. All subjects underwent transcranial Doppler after injection of agitated saline into the antecubital vein to look for evidence of right-to-left intracardiac shunting. As in the first study, measurements were taken during normal breathing and after a Valsalva maneuver. The appearance of microbubbles in the brain vessels within 7 seconds was considered a positive study. A PFO was present in 48% of patients with migraine headache with aura, compared with only 23% of patients with migraine headache without aura and 20% of age-matched controls. The difference in PFO prevalence between the aura-positive group and the aura-negative group was statistically significant (odds ratio [OR], 3.13; 95% CI, 1.41–7.04; $P = 0.002$), as was the difference between the aura-positive group and the control group (OR, 3.66; 95% CI, 1.21–13.25; $P = 0.01$). There was not a statistically significant difference between the migraine headache without aura group and the controls (OR,

1.17; 95% CI, 0.32–4.45; $P =$ not significant). This study provides further evidence of a link between migraine headache with aura and PFO.

A third study examining the link between PFO and migraine headache is that of Wilmshurst and Nightingale [12]. This British group has done extensive work with divers who have experienced decompression sickness, and throughout this work they have noted that there seemed to be a correlation between migraine headache with aura in daily life and a large right-to-left shunt. They performed a case series of 200 divers who had been referred for decompression sickness, in which all patients underwent transthoracic echocardiography including injection of agitated saline through the antecubital vein to look for an intracardiac right-to-left shunt. As in the studies previously described, the procedure was performed during normal breathing and after a Valsalva maneuver. They classified patients according to migraine headache with aura in daily life (ie, activities unconnected with diving), migraine headache without aura in daily life, and no migraine headaches in daily life. The authors found intra-atrial shunting in 53% of cases (106/200), and these shunts were graded as small (12 cases), medium (5 cases), or large (89 cases); if large, they were further categorized as present only with Valsalva or present at rest. There was not a statistically significant difference between the presence or size of a shunt and the prevalence rate of migraine headache without aura in daily life. Patients with a large shunt at rest, however, were significantly more likely to have migraine headache with aura (38/80, 47.5%) than were patients with any other size of shunt, including those with a large shunt present during Valsalva (15/120, 12.5%) ($P < 0.001$; OR and 95% CI not provided). These findings suggest that there is an association between migraine headache with aura and the presence of a large, continuously present right-to-left intracardiac shunt.

The Patent Foramen Ovale and Atrial Septal Aneurism study examined the prevalence of migraine headache in a cohort of 581 young patients with cryptogenic stroke (Table 2) [13]. Unlike the studies previously described, this study diagnosed PFO using transthoracic echocardiography. If three or more microbubbles were seen in the left atrium within three cardiac cycles, with or without Valsalva maneuver, the study was considered positive for PFO. In this cohort the prevalence of migraine headache was nearly double among those with a PFO versus those without: migraine headache was present in 27% of patients with PFO versus 14% of patients without a PFO (OR, 1.75; 95% CI, 1.08–2.82; $P = 0.0001$).

Sztajzel et al (see Table 2) [14] reported similar findings in a case series of 74 patients with acute stroke of undetermined origin. PFOs were diagnosed using transcranial Doppler and were found in 44 of the 74 patients; of these, 16 (36%) reported a history of migraine headache with aura. In the 30 patients in the series without PFO, only 4 patients (13%) reported a history of migraine headache with aura, a statistically significant difference ($P = 0.03$; OR and CI not provided). Furthermore, of 44 patients with PFO, the intracardiac shunt was thought to play a causal role in the stroke in 25 patients. Of these 25 patients, 13 (52%) reported migraine headache with aura, compared with only 3 (16%) of the patients who were believed not to have a causal PFO-stroke relationship ($P = 0.014$; OR and CI not provided).

Positive effect of patent foramen ovale closure on migraine headache

These studies show a statistically significant higher prevalence of PFO in patients who suffer from migraine headache with aura. If there is a causal relationship between the presence of PFO and migraine headache with (or without) aura, closure of a patient's PFO should result in resolution of or decreased intensity and frequency of migraine headaches. The following studies attempt to answer that question. Wilmshurst

and colleagues [15] followed up on their 1999 study of PFO prevalence in divers with migraine headache with a retrospective study in 2000 looking at the effect of intracardiac shunt closure on migraine headaches. They studied 37 patients who had undergone intracardiac shunt closure to permit resumption of diving after decompression illness, after stroke, or to close a large defect. Of those patients, 21 had reported migraine headache before closure (16 with aura and 5 without). None of the closures were performed because of migraine headache, and the patients were not given any reason to expect that migraine headache symptoms would improve after closure of their intracardiac defect. In long-term follow-up, 10 of the 21 patients (7 with aura and 3 without) had complete resolution of their migraine headaches. Eight additional patients (all of whom had migraine headache with aura) reported improvement in severity and frequency of their migraine headaches. This study has the potential drawback of being purely retrospective and therefore subject to reporting bias.

Morandi et al [16] report a case series of 17 migraine headache patients undergoing percutaneous transcatheter closure of a PFO after suffering a cryptogenic stroke. Patients were asked to report retrospectively the intensity, frequency, duration, and presence or absence of aura of their migraine headaches for the 3 months preceding their transcatheter closure. They were then given a diary to record prospective symptoms over the next 6 months. Of the 17 patients, 8 suffered from migraine headache with aura, and 9 had migraine headache without aura. After percutaneous shunt closure, there was a statistically significant decrease in the number of bubbles seen in the cranial circulation on subsequent transcranial Doppler studies and in the severity (frequency, duration, and intensity) of migraine headaches at 1-, 3-, and 6-month follow-up ($P = 0.0002$, $P = 0.0002$, and $P = 0.0008$ at 1, 3, and 6 months, respectively, versus baseline data; OR and CI not provided).

Table 2
Prevalence of migraines in patients with patent foramen ovale detected in the workup of a stroke evaluation

Study	Total # of patients	% of PFO patients with migraine	% non-PFO patients with migraine	Odds ratio	95% confidence interval	P
Patent Foramen Ovale and Atrial Septal Aneurism Study Group, 2002	581	27%	14%	1.75	1.08-2.82	0.0001
Stajzel, 2002	74	16/36 (36%)	4/30 (13%)			0.03

Migraine headaches completely ceased in 5 patients, and were substantially improved in 10. Morandi et al [16] did not find a statistical difference between improvement in the migraine headache with aura group and the migraine headache without aura group, but the study size was quite small.

A Swiss study from 2004 looked at a series of 215 patients undergoing percutaneous closure of PFO after presumed paradoxical embolism [17]. In this cohort, 22% of patients reported at least one migraine headache in the year before closure, an incidence that the authors report is twice the incidence of migraine headache in the general European population. In the subgroup of patients with aura-positive migraine headache, PFO closure resulted in a 54% reduction in the frequency of migraine headache attacks ($P = 0.001$). Similarly, among aura-negative migraine headache patients in the cohort, PFO closure resulted in a 62% decrease in the frequency of migraine headaches ($P = 0.006$). Patients in the cohort with headaches that did not meet migraine headache criteria did not have a significant change in headache frequency after PFO closure.

Negative effect of closure of intracardiac shunt on migraine headache

Two cases have been reported of an intra-atrial shunt closure resulting in transformation from intermittent migraine headache into daily migraine headache. An important distinction however, is that in both these cases the interatrial shunting was through a relatively large atrial septal defect (ASD), not a PFO. Yankovsky and Kuritzky [18] report a 48-year-old man who underwent routine closure of a 26-mm ASD. He had suffered from migraine headache with aura intermittently since age 13 years. After closure of the ASD with an Amplatzer device (AGA Medical Corporation, Golden Valley, Minnesota), he began to experience daily migraine headache with aura, which continued for 6 months, always starting at 11 A.M. A follow-up transesophageal echocardiogram verified that there was no residual shunting, and no other cause could be found based on that study. After 6 months, the migraine headaches decreased in frequency from daily to weekly, and after propranolol prophylaxis was begun, he finally became nearly asymptomatic. Rodes-Cabau et al [19] report a case of a percutaneous ASD closure in a 31-year-old woman that resulted in new-onset migraine headache. The patient underwent closure

after routine discovery of a significant left-to-right shunt, and she had no history of migraine headache. Thirty-six hours after closure, she began to have photopsia, left-sided scotoma, pulsating head pain, photophobia, phonophobia, nausea, vomiting, and paresthesia in the left hand and leg. Several subsequent attacks followed in the next week and then decreased in frequency without treatment in the following weeks. The attacks persisted intermittently for 3 months, at which time amitriptyline treatment was initiated, and the attacks stopped. Imaging, including a brain CT, brain MRI, transcranial Doppler imaging, and transesophageal echocardiography, was negative for emboli, and the device was confirmed to be in the correct position.

In their 2000 article Wilmshurst and colleagues [15] reported that 11 of the patients undergoing closure of a PFO noted fortification spectra immediately after closure, and 4 of these patients had typical migraine headaches immediately after closure as well, indicating that migraine headache immediately after closure is not rare. In the same study, one patient noted new splinter hemorrhages in her fingernails in the week immediately following shunt closure.

Comment

The correlation between PFO closure and a decrease in migraine headache severity and frequency supports multiple theories of migraine headache pathogenesis, including a causative role for paradoxical microemboli to the terminal branches of the basovertebral artery. Additionally, an intracardiac shunt could allow vasoactive substances such as atrial natriuretic peptide (ANP), platelet factors, and amines to bypass the pulmonary filter, triggering migraine headache [12]. Some of the studies in this article noted a decrease in frequency of migraine headache with aura as well as migraine headache without aura after shunt closure. This finding could be explained by the theory that migraine headache without aura is similar physiologically to migraine headache with aura, except that the circulation involved affects silent areas of cortex rather than visual, motor, or sensory cortex.

If paradoxical microemboli are responsible for migraine headache with aura, closing a PFO should improve the frequency of attacks, if not eliminate them. The experience in at least two patients of new-onset or worsening pattern of migraine headache attacks does not fit the theory as easily. Both of these cases involved closure of an ASD, not a PFO. This distinction is important because ASDs typically shunt predominantly from left to right, and PFOs shunt predominantly from right to left. The authors of that study note that transesophageal echo and transcranial Doppler showed no evidence of embolic events, and there did not seem to be any clot forming on the catheter. As is standard practice, the patient was receiving antiplatelet therapy, making platelet aggregation or factor activation an unlikely cause of migraine headache. They propose that stretching of the left atrium with the device in place could release ANP, which has been proposed as one of the vasoactive substances potentially responsible for the pathogenesis of migraine headache. Clearly, closing a large ASD does suddenly expose the left atrium to an additional volume and would result in some stretching.

To date, the body of evidence linking PFO and migraine headaches is limited but intriguing, hindered by small patient numbers and nonuniformity of study methods. Most studies have used transcranial Doppler to diagnose PFO; this modality is generally held to be the most sensitive but not the most specific method of diagnosing a PFO. Transesophageal echocardiogram is the most specific method but is less sensitive than transcranial Doppler; no study used this method. One study used transthoracic echo, which is considered to have a lower sensitivity and specificity than either of the other methods. Additionally, the criteria used for defining a positive study differ among the studies, varying in both the number of microbubbles in circulation and the length of time when they are seen. Finally, some studies do not distinguish in their data analyses between migraine headache with and without aura; those that make this distinction show a much stronger correlation between migraine headache with aura and PFO than between migraine headache without aura and PFO.

The argument for PFO as a causal agent in migraine headache is lacking in at least one important respect: closing a PFO does not completely cure migraine headaches in all patients, and not all migraine headache patients have been found to have an intracardiac shunt (or atrial septal aneurysm). There are two plausible explanations for these observations. Perhaps PFOs (or other intracardiac shunts) were missed in some migraine headache patients in these studies because of the lower sensitivity of injection of agitated saline into the antecubital vein instead

of the femoral vein (the femoral vein has a higher sensitivity because bubbles entering the atrium from the inferior vena cava have a trajectory different from that of bubbles entering from the superior vena cava) [20,21]. Femoral vein injection increases the sensitivity by only a few percentage points, however. More migraine headache is multifactorial, and for some patients, closing a PFO is not sufficient to eradicate the migraine headaches; conversely, a PFO is not sufficient by itself in some patients to cause migraine headache, explaining the lack of a one-to-one relationship.

Despite the relative safety of the transcatheter closure procedure, it seems imprudent, based on the above evidence, to recommend PFO closure as a first-line treatment for migraine headache. Indeed, given the lack of universal improvement in patients suffering from migraines with PFO closure, no patients should be given the hope that PFO closure would help their migraines. For patients with migraine and PFO who have other clear reasons for closing the PFO, the expectation should be that migraines may improve, but most likely there will be no effect. Likewise, it should not be an expectation that migraines will worsen with PFO closure, because evidence to this effect seems largely anecdotal to date. It does seem evident; however, that PFO plays a convincing role in the pathogenesis of migraine headache in some individuals.

References

[1] Headache Classification Subcommittee of the International Headache Society. The international classification of headache disorders, 2nd edition. Cephalalgia 2004;24(Suppl. 1):1–36.

[2] Stewart WF, Lipton RB, Liberman J. Variation in migraine prevalence by race. Neurology 1996;47(1): 52–9.

[3] Osterhaus JT, Gutterman DL, Plachetka JR. Healthcare resource and lost labor costs of migraine headache in the US. Pharmacoeconomics 1992;2: 67–76.

[4] Clouse JC, Osterhaus JT. Healthcare resource use and costs associated with migraine in a managed healthcare setting. Ann Pharmacother 1994;28: 659–64.

[5] Headache Classification Committee of the International Headache Society. Classification and diagnostic criteria for headache disorders, cranial neuralgias and facial pain. Cephalalgia 1988;8(Suppl 7):1–96.

[6] Carolei A, Marini C, De Matteis G, and the Italian National Research Council Study Group on Stroke in the Young. History of migraine and risk of cerebral ischemia in young adults. Lancet 1996;347:1503–6.

[7] Tzourio C, Tehindrazanarivelo A, Iglesias S, et al. Case-control study of migraine and risk of ischemic stroke in young women BMJ 1995;310: 830–3.

[8] Overell JR, Bone I, Lees KR. Interatrial septal abnormalities and stroke: a meta-analysis of case-control studies Neurology 2000;55:1172–9.

[9] Hagen PT, Scholz DG, Edwards WD. Incidence and size of patent foramen ovale during the first 10 decades of life: an autopsy study of 965 normal hearts. Mayo Clin Proc 1984;59:17–20.

[10] Del Sette M, Angeli S, Leandri M, et al. Migraine with aura and right-to-left shunt on transcranial Doppler: a case-control study. Cerebrovasc Dis 1998;8(6):327–30.

[11] Anzola GP, Mangoni M, Guindani M, et al. Potential source of cerebral embolism in migraine with aura: a transcranial Doppler study. Neurology 1999;52:1622–5.

[12] Wilmshurst P, Nightingale S. Relationship between migraine and cardiac and pulmonary right-to-left shunts. Clin Sci 2001;100:215–20.

[13] Lamy C, Giannesini C, Zuber M, for the Patent Foramen Ovale and Atrial Septal Aneurism Study Group. Clinical and imaging findings in cryptogenic stroke patients with and without patent foramen ovale. The PFO-ASA Study. Stroke 2002;33: 706–11.

[14] Sztajzel R, Genoud D, Roth S, et al. Patent foramen ovale, a possible cause of symptomatic migraine: a study of 74 patients with acute ischemic stroke. Cerebrovasc Dis 2002;13:102–6.

[15] Wilmshurst PT, Nightingale S, Walsh KP, et al. Effect on migraine of closure of cardiac right-to-left shunts to prevent recurrence of decompression illness or stroke or for hemodynamic reasons. Lancet 2000;356:1648–51.

[16] Morandi E, Anzola GP, Angeli S, et al. Transcatheter closure of patent foramen ovale: a new migraine treatment? J Interv Cardiol 2003;16:39–42.

[17] Schwerzmann M, Wiher S, Nedeltchev K, et al. Percutaneous closure of patent foramen ovale reduces the frequency of migraine attacks. Neurology 2004; 62:1399–401.

[18] Yankovsky AE, Kuritzky A. Transformation into daily migraine with aura following transcutaneous atrial septal defect closure. Headache 2003;42: 496–8.

[19] Rodes-Cabau J, Molina C, Serrano-Munuera C, et al. Migraine with aura related to the percutaneous closure of an atrial septal defect. Catheter Cardiovasc Interv 2003;60:540–2.

[20] Gin KG, Huckell VF, Pollick C. Femoral vein delivery of contrast medium enhances transthoracic echocardiographic detection of patent foramen ovale. J Am Coll Cardiol 1993;22:1994–2000.

[21] Hamann GF, Schatzer-Klotz D, Frohlig G, et al. Femoral injection of echo contrast medium may increase the sensitivity of testing for a patent foramen ovale. Neurology 1998;50:1423–8.

ELSEVIER
SAUNDERS

Cardiol Clin 23 (2005) 97–104

CARDIOLOGY
CLINICS

Patent Foramen Ovale and Diving

Peter Germonpré, MD

Centre for Hyperbaric Oxygen Therapy, Military Hospital Brussels, Bruynstraat 200, Brussels 1120, Belgium

Diving using self-contained underwater breathing apparatus (SCUBA) has gained an enormous popularity over the last 20 years and has evolved from a "macho" sport toward an activity accessible to all. Worldwide, more than 10 million people engage in sports diving and annually, on estimate, more than 250 million dives are performed [1].

Although SCUBA diving is perceived as a high-risk sport by insurance companies and by the general public, it is generally safe. Because the majority of accidents are related to cardiac pathology and drowning, good health and a proper medical check-up are essential in reducing the risks. The most dreaded accidents, however, are related to so-called "decompression disorders," in part because their origin and exact cause is not always clearly understood.

A complete review of decompression-related diseases is beyond the scope of this article, but a brief overview of the pathophysiology of decompression sickness and barotrauma is presented here.

In compliance with the physical gas laws, air, or any other inhaled gas, is compressed as the diver descends under water. The volume of any gas body decreases proportionally with increasing pressure and expands again upon ascent from depth (Boyle's Law) if no gas molecules are added or removed. Gas molecules are dissolved in the tissue fluids proportionally to the ambient pressure, and inert gases, such as nitrogen, need to be expired again when the diver ascends (Henry's Law). The speed and extent of this saturation depends primarily on the depth (pressure) and the time spent at depth but is also influenced by other so-called "personal" factors, such as cardiac output, local perfusion, pulmonary diffusion coefficient, and body fat percentage [2].

At the end of the dive, care must be taken not to ascend (ie, reduce the ambient pressure) too quickly. If the pressure differential is too great, there is a risk that nitrogen will come out of solution already in the blood stream, and form nitrogen bubbles (venous gas emboli [VGE]). The site of generation of these bubbles is at the venous end of the capillary bed, at the outflow of the saturated tissues. These bubbles may stay locally trapped, causing no symptoms, or, when bigger, may cause local ischemia or pain. Alternately, they may be released into the venous blood stream and transported into the central venous bed. Unless the bubble load is very high, these VGE are temporarily trapped in the pulmonary capillary bed and disappear after some minutes by the diffusion of nitrogen (the lung is an excellent bubble filter capable of eliminating all but the most severe postdive VGE occurrences) [3,4]. When bubbles do pass the pulmonary filter [5], they become arterial gas emboli and may cause ischemic lesions at the site where they are finally trapped. All symptoms caused by decompression bubbles, whether local, venous, or arterial, are classified under the term "decompression sickness" (DCS) [6].

To prevent decompression sickness, decompression algorithms (dive tables) have been developed, originally by military organizations and later by commercial and civilian dive organizations. These algorithms impose "decompression stops" at certain depths for a certain time to allow the nitrogen partial pressure in the body to be reduced to a level where decompression can safely be resumed. Based on a purely observational model, over the years these algorithms have

E-mail address: peter.germonpre@mil.be

become complex mathematical models, taking into account several body compartments, each with different saturation-desaturation speeds [7–9]. They have been incorporated in wrist-worn dive computers and generally perform well in preventing decompression sickness [10].

These decompression algorithms have always used clinical DCS as an end-point for evaluating their effectiveness. This procedure of course maximizes the available safe "bottom time," which is the primary purpose of decompression algorithms. It has been shown, however, that after many, if not most, deeper dives (25–30 meters of sea water [msw] or deeper) with obligatory decompression stops, VGE are present in different degrees in many divers [2,11,12]. There is an important inter- and intra-individual variation in the degree of bubbling after a dive, indicating a large influence of the personal factors affecting saturation and desaturation. Although in most cases these VGE do not lead to decompression sickness, they can be the cause of so-called "unexplained DCS" [13].

History of diving accidents related to patent foramen ovale

Although paradoxical embolism through a patent foramen ovale (PFO) had been described as early as in 1877 [14], and paradoxical gas embolism was described in 1979 [15], the first reports of a possible relationship between decompression sickness and patency of the foramen ovale date only from 1989 [16]. Since then, considerable controversy has arisen concerning the real importance of PFO as a risk factor for diving. This controversy is related to several factors.

First, the diagnosis of decompression sickness is by no means easy, and vague or minor symptoms are often neglected or overlooked by the diver [17] or by the medical team. On the other hand, neurologic symptoms after a dive may be caused by pathologic conditions not related to decompression, such as neck hyperextension, or even to illness not related to diving [18,19]. Therefore, the exact incidence of decompression sickness is unknown.

Second, it is generally assumed by the diver and the medical team that, if the diver has committed errors in the decompression process (eg, by performing a rapid ascent or by omitting some or all of the prescribed decompression stops), the decompression sickness is around deserved, that is, it would have occurred whether the foramen ovale was patent or not. Any increase of the DCS risk by the PFO is thus ignored.

Third, the techniques used for detecting and evaluating PFO are by no means standardized. The reference standard for detecting PFO using contrast transesophageal echocardiography (c-TEE), is itself defined equivocally, and variations in technique have led to a large inter- and intra-observer variability. Prevalences as low as 9% to as high as 40% have been reported in a representative sample of a normal population [20,21], whereas the anatomic prevalence is known to be around 25% [22,23]. Other indirect techniques have a lower sensibility (transthoracic echocardiography [TTE]) or detect right-to-left shunts reliably but cannot distinguish between PFO and extracardiac (pulmonary) shunts (transcranial Doppler [TCD]) [24]. Therefore, the exact prevalence of PFO in divers with decompression sickness is not known with certainty. The authors have repeatedly stressed the importance of a proper standardization of the c-TEE technique, more specifically of standardizing the straining maneuver used, and of completely describing the technique used in each research report [25,26].

Considerable attention has been given recently to the possibility of subclinical cerebral damage by caused by repeated embolization of gas emboli through a PFO after each dive. These studies rely mainly on MRI data and indicate a possible higher incidence of cerebral white matter lesions in divers with PFO, even if they have never suffered from DCS [27,28]. These findings raise great concerns among divers, because, if they were confirmed, PFO could represent a major long-term risk factor in diving [29]. Most of these studies, however, suffer from a number of methodologic errors, ranging from selection bias (divers who have suffered cerebral DCS but were never treated because of denial or ignorance might self-select for evaluation), over population inadequacy (some studies mix professional and sports divers, of a wide age range and with dive experience ranging from 5 to 2000 dives), to technical methodologic errors (eg, in PFO detection or inadequate MR technique). Furthermore, the nature of these white matter lesions has not been proven to be vascular [30], and their presence is seldom correlated with functional neuropsychometric alterations.

Retrospective evidence of increased risk with patent foramen ovale

Retrospective studies compare divers who have suffered from DCS with healthy volunteers, both divers or nondivers. Divers with neurologic DCS were found to have a significantly higher prevalence of PFO (Table 1). From these retrospective studies, the odds ratio (OR) can be calculated for the probability of suffering DCS when diving with a PFO. From a combined analysis of the c-TTE studies, an OR of 2.6 has been calculated. The c-TEE and c-TCD studies yielded ORs of 5.6 [25], 4.3 [36], and 4.8 [59], respectively.

Nature of decompression pathology related to patent foramen ovale

PFO-related decompression sickness is presumed to be caused by paradoxical nitrogen bubble embolization through the interatrial septum. After many long, deep (25 msw or more) dives, large numbers of nitrogen microbubbles (19–700 microns in diameter) [4] can be detected in the central venous circulation. If about 25% of all divers have a PFO, why does this condition not lead to decompression sickness more often?

It is a popular misconception that a PFO allows the continuous passage of blood between the right and the left atrium. Although a PFO is a right-to-left shunt, flow characteristics in the heart are such that this passage rarely occurs.

First, during 95% of the cardiac cycle, the atrial pressure on the right side of the heart is lower than on the left side. Because the foramen ovale is a valvelike structure opening from right to left, this pressure differential tends to close the valve, prohibiting passage of blood and bubbles [31]. Second, the flow coming from the superior vena cava passes over a tissue fold of the right atrial wall before reaching the fossa ovalis. Passage over this fold causes a sudden increase in the rate of the flow, and when this flow meets the flow coming from the inferior vena cava, it causes a venous turbulence in the right atrium. This turbulence tends to sweep blood from the inferior vena cava (where most of the bubbles

arise after a dive) away from the interatrial septum [32]. Under normal conditions these two mechanisms would prohibit venous blood and bubbles from crossing the foramen ovale.

After diving, however, two other conditions may arise to facilitate or permit this right-to-left shunt. Continuous pulmonary embolization of nitrogen microbubbles invariably leads to increased pulmonary vascular resistance and, retrogradely, to increased right atrial pressure. This augmentation may increase the right atrial pressure above the left atrial pressure for sufficient time to allow shunting of blood [33]. Also, as can be demonstrated during c-TEE, certain respiratory maneuvers, by varying the intrathoracic pressure, may temporarily reverse the interatrial pressure gradient and thus permit shunting. These maneuvers can be voluntary or involuntary [31,34]. A typical example in diving is lifting of heavy air tanks into the boat or car trunk or climbing aboard a Zodiac craft or raft. Bubbles are present in the venous blood for up to 2 hours after surfacing [11], making these maneuvers typical circumstances of PFO-related DCS.

After right-to-left shunting, these arterialized bubbles follow the predominant course of blood flow into the aortic cross and further into the cerebral circulation. Upright posture facilitates this passage into the cerebrum because of the natural tendency of bubbles to float upwards in a liquid. The pathway from VGE to cerebral arterial gas embolism has been demonstrated clearly by TCD in sports divers after a dive: the number of bubbles detectable in the middle cerebral artery was proportional to the degree of patency of the foramen ovale [35].

In fact, nitrogen decompression bubbles then act as arterial gas emboli, and one would expect symptoms similar to those of iatrogenic gas embolization.

Early reports established a possible relationship between PFO and neurologic, early-onset

Table 1
Retrospective studies

Reference	PFO prevalence (%) in neurologic DCS divers (n)	PFO prevalence (%) in controls (n)	Type of controls	Technique used
Moon et al 1989 [16]	61.1 (301)	10.8 (176)	Nonmatched nondivers	c-TTE
Wilmshurst et al 1989 [57]	66 (61)	24 (63)	Nonmatched divers	c-TTE
Kerut et al 1997 [58]	60 (26)	47 (30)	Matched nondivers	c-TEE
Germonpré et al 1998 [25]	59.9 (37)	36.1 (36)	Matched divers	c-TEE
Cantais et al 2003 [36]	58.4 (101)	24.8 (101)	Nonmatched divers	c-TCD
Torti et al 2004 [59]	64 (28)	25.7 (175)	Nonmatched divers	c-TEE

DCS (occurring less than 30 minutes after the dive). This association is consistent with the proposed pathophysiologic mechanism of shunting [16,31]. Later, a relationship between PFO and cerebral or high-spinal (but not low-spinal) DCS became apparent, confirming the proposed preferential pathway of the bubbles [36–38].

PFO-related DCS, then, seems characterized by

- Early onset (within 30 minutes to 1 hour after surfacing from a saturating dive) [39]
- A dive performed in accordance with the currently accepted decompression algorithms (although violation of those rules obviously produces even more microbubbles) [25]
- Neurologic symptoms pointing to a cerebral, cerebellar, ocular, vestibular, auditory, or high-spinal lesion, rather than joint pains, lymphatic obstruction, or a lower spinal syndrome [36, 38,40]

The association between this "undeserved cerebral DCS" and PFO seems solidly proven: by both c-TEE and c-TCD, up to 80% of these divers have been shown to be PFO positive [25,36].

Somewhat puzzling is the strong association that has been suggested between PFO and cutaneous symptoms of DCS—painful red-blue stripes on thorax, shoulders, and abdomen (cutis marmorata) [41,42]. In contrast with the classical description of cutaneous DCS, however, these lesions do not exhibit subcutaneous crepitations, nor are they necessarily localized on areas of local blood flow obstruction [42]. Therefore, it seems more justified and pathophysiologically sound to consider them manifestations of a central nervous system (brainstem) embolization rather than as a local phenomenon. (The clinical picture is similar to the cutis marmorata commonly seen in newborn infants, where it is a manifestation of an immature autonomic nervous system) [43,44]. For obvious ethical reasons, this hypothesis has not been and would be impossible to prove in a human experimental model.

Prospective evaluation of increased risk

One reason why not more of the divers with PFO are affected by neurologic DCS may be the "fast-tissue" nature of the brain; that is, the brain has a sufficiently high and constant blood supply so that it can desaturate quickly after a dive [45]. By the time nitrogen bubbles actually are embolized into the brain (20 to 30 minutes after surfacing from the dive), the partial nitrogen pressure in brain tissue would probably be sufficiently low for nitrogen to diffuse out of the bubble rapidly. Therefore, the bubble would shrink and disappear without causing any damage. No DCS would result [39].

This process would also explain why vestibular/auditory DCS often appears as an isolated phenomenon, without other apparent symptoms of cerebral DCS. Indeed, for bubbles to embolize the inferior anterior cerebellar artery and reach the vestibular apparatus [46], a large number of bubbles need to pass into the basilar artery. Because the brain (a fast tissue) is far more desaturated than the vestibular system (a slow tissue) and has a far better collateral circulation, cerebral bubbles disappear quickly, and symptoms arise only in the vestibular apparatus. A similar mechanism may also be the reason why fewer cases of purely cerebral DCS (symptoms pointing to frontal and middle lobes) have been described than cases of posterior cerebral, cerebellar, and brainstem DCS.

When only clinical DCS is taken into consideration, and possible diagnostic errors caused by vague and minor symptoms are disregarded, the risk of a diver's incurring DCS is low. According to statistics by the Divers Alert Network Europe [47], one DCS occurs for every 6400 dives deeper than 30 msw. One DCS occurs per 43,000 dives if only dives shallower than 30 msw are counted. Other diver and dive-safety organizations report similar incidence rates for DCS [48,49]. The calculation of an odds ratio of the order of 4 to 6 justifies a prospective study on PFO and DCS. This study, using a carotid Doppler screening method for determining right-to-left shunts, is ongoing but will probably not be completed until about 2010 [50].

Changing patency over time

Finally, when making statements about the risk of PFO for divers, one must take into account the possibility that a PFO may evolve over time and possibly become more patent after some years.

In the classical autopsy studies performed in 1931 and 1984 [22,23], different age cohorts seemed to have different patency prevalence (Table 2). This finding suggests that PFOs tend to close with advancing age unless they are large or unless something keeps them open.

Table 2
PFO prevalence in different age cohorts: autopsy data

Author	1–20 Years (%)	20–40 Years (%)	>40 Years (%)
Patten 1931 [23]	34.5	27.2	22.4
Hagen 1984 [22]	35	29	20.4

Anecdotal observations of divers who, after an uneventful diving career of many years, suddenly seemed to become extremely susceptible to DCS with the comorbid observation of a large PFO [51] prompted the author and colleagues to investigate whether, over time, the prevalence or size of PFO is subject to change among divers.

A group of 40 divers who had undergone investigation for PFO, using a strictly standardized technique of c-TEE in the period from 1994 to 1996, gave their informed consent for a re-evaluation using the same technique, 6 to 8 years later. Ethics committee approval was obtained for this follow-up echocardiographic study. The group consisted of 40 divers, of whom 16 had suffered DCS previously and 24 had never experienced DCS but had served as matched controls for the initial study. All divers had continued diving and had not suffered DCS since their first c-TEE.

Patency of the foramen ovale was assessed with a highly standardized c-TEE technique, as described earlier [25]. PFOs were semiquantitatively graded as grade 0 (no bubble passage), grade I (less than 20 bubbles), or grade II (large patency, more than 20 bubbles).

To exclude enhanced detection of PFO as compared with the initial tests performed several

years earlier, the following precautions were taken:

- The examining cardiologist was blinded to the initial c-TEE result
- Contrast-enhancing features of the TEE system (harmonic imaging) were not used [52]
- The sequence of the c-TEE examination, as described in the original study protocol, was repeated meticulously, even if during everyday c-TEE examinations, the cardiologists might have used other techniques to improve detection of PFO

The initial prevalence of PFO in this group of divers was 50% (20/40), of whom 9 (22.5% of total) had a grade I and 11 (27.5% of total) had a grade II PFO. Mean years of diving between the two c-TEEs was 7.19, and the mean number of dives was 286 (mean, 39 dives/y). The final prevalence of PFO was 52.5% (21/40).

Of the 20 divers who initially presented without a PFO, 3 were found to have a grade I PFO after a mean of 7.6 years and 556 dives. One diver had a grade II PFO (after 7 years, 150 dives). Sixteen divers were still grade 0 (mean, 7.24 years; 279 dives).

Of the 9 divers with an initial grade I PFO, 5 divers were found to have a grade II PFO after a mean of 7.54 years and 218 dives. Three divers with a former PFO were found to be contrast negative (7.04 years; 217 dives) (Table 3).

The difference of c-TEE score on an ordinal scale was statistically significant (Wilcoxon signed rank test; $P = 0.0354$). Using a Friedman 1-way ANOVA by ranks, this difference approached

Table 3
Longitudinal survey of patent foramen ovale in divers (mean: 7 years)

PFO grade	c-TEE 1 n (%)	Evolution Grade	n	Years/Dives	c-TEE 2 n (%)
Grade 0	20 (50)	0	16	7.24/279	19 (47.5)
		I	3	7.68/557	
		II	1	7.0/150	
Grade I		0	3	7.04/217	4 (10)
	9 (22.5)	I	1	5/450	
		II	5	7.54/218	
Grade II		0	0		17 (42.5)
		II	0		
	11 (27.5)	II	11	7.15/325	
Total	40				40

Data from Germonpre P, Balestra C, Unger P, et al. Time-related opening of the foramen ovale in divers. In: Germonpre P, Balestra C, editors. Proceedings of the 28th Annual Meeting of the European Underwater and Baromedical Society, 2002. Bruges (Belgium): ACHOBEL (Advisory Committee for Hyperbaric Oxygen in Belgium);2002.

significance ($P = 0.0833$, chi-square approximation with correction for ties). This study [60]
showed that over a period of 7 years, the permeability of the foramen ovale in a group of sports
divers was changing in both directions, towards
closure in 7.5% of the divers and towards increased permeability in 22.5% (half of whom—
10%—had no initial permeability).

The findings in this small series, with prospective assessment are consistent with the findings in different age groups by autopsy studies.

To the author's knowledge, this study was the
first prospective follow-up study using essentially
the same and reliable technique to document an
increase in PFO size in sports divers. This finding
may suggest that divers could develop an increased
susceptibility for neurologic DCS over time and
may explain the observation that experienced
divers who had never suffered DCS in their many
years of diving are diagnosed with an unexplain-
ably large PFO after their first episode of DCS.

A novel finding was that four divers who were
PFO-negative in the initial study 7 years previously presented with PFO in this study. It may
be suggested that finding merely reflects an increased detection rate resulting from the use of
more powerful equipment, a more optimized
examination technique, or more experienced cardiologists. The author and colleagues anticipated
this criticism by deliberately "downscaling" their
detection technique to obtain images of the same
quality as in the initial study. Moreover, the
cardiologists (already experienced in the initial
study) were blinded to the result of the initial tests.
Third, as in the initial study, the images were
evaluated independently by all cardiologists involved. Therefore, the author and colleagues
believe that this finding was not an artifact.

It is possible that the fusion of the interatrial
septum was incomplete in these divers from the
onset. No contrast passage could be shown during
the initial c-TEE examination, indicating either
a complete closure or minimal (microscopic)
opening of the interatrial valve. If the latter had
been the case, the total number of divers with
"increased permeability of PFO" would be 9
(22.5%). This finding also would be important
and a cause for concern, because it would suggest
that many (more than half) of divers with a grade
I PFO could eventually develop a grade II PFO
and thus incur a statistically significant increased
risk for neurologic DCS. Incidentally, a recent
study that examined a random sample of experienced divers who had never suffered from DCS

found a PFO prevalence of 65%, with a grade II
PFO in 38% in these divers [53].

Mechanisms for de novo opening of PFOs
could involve diving-related phenomena, such as
variations in the right atrial pressures during the
end stages of dives [33,54] or events immediately
following, a dive. Such fluctuations in pressure are
equally associated with straining-release events
such as those encountered in certain types of
exercise and in activities of daily living [34,55]. No
specific diving-related hypothesis is suggested at
this time.

Summary

Patency of the foramen ovale is a risk factor
for DCS in SCUBA divers, even if they adhere to
the currently accepted and used decompression
tables. The primary cause of DCS, however, is the
nitrogen bubble, not the PFO. There are a number
of techniques any diver can use to minimize the
occurrence of nitrogen bubbles after a dive.

The authors current practice is to inform
civilian sports divers of the increased risk and to
advise them to adopt conservative dive profiles.
This can be achieved by selecting a more conservative dive computer, performing only dives that
do not require obligatory decompression stops, or
using oxygen-enriched breathing gas mixtures
("nitrox") while still diving on "air profiles" [56].

Dive-safety organizations are currently under-
taking studies aimed at proposing changes in the
decompression algorithms to produce low-bubble
dive tables [12]. In the meantime, PFO remains
a reason for caution.

Whether all divers should be screened for PFO
is an ongoing discussion [50] in view of methodologic and practical issues outlined in this article.
Any definitive recommendations can be made
only after a careful, prospective evaluation of
the real relative risk for DCS and long-term
cerebral damage.

References

[1] Scuba diving. In: UN atlas of the oceans. Available
    at: Web Encyclopedia, http://www.oceansatlas.org.
    2002. Accessed September 1, 2004.
[2] Carturan D, Boussuges A, Vanuxem P, et al. Ascent
    rate, age, maximal oxygen uptake, adiposity, and
    circulating venous bubbles after diving. J Appl Phys-
    iol 2002;93(4):1349–56.
[3] Butler BD, Hills BA. The lung as a filter for micro-
    bubbles. J Appl Physiol 1979;47(3):537–43.

[4] Hills BA, Butler BD. Size distribution of intravascular air emboli produced by decompression. Undersea Biomed Res 1981;8(3):163–70.

[5] Niden AH, Aviado DM. Effects of pulmonary embolism on the pulmonary circulation with special reference to arteriovenous shunts in the lung. Circ Res 1956;4:67–73.

[6] Moon RE. Classification of the decompression disorders: time to accept reality. Undersea Hyperb Med 1997;24(1):2–4.

[7] Yount DE, Hoffman DC. On the use of a bubble formation model to calculate diving tables. Aviat Space Environ Med 1986;57(2):149–56.

[8] Yarbrough OD. Calculation of decompression tables. Research report. Washington, DC: US Navy Experimental Diving Unit; 1937.

[9] Boycott AE, Damant GC, Haldane JS. The prevention of compressed-air illness. J Hygiene 1908;8:342–443.

[10] Acott CJ. Diving incident monitoring study: dive tables and dive computers. SPUMS J 1994;24(4):214–5.

[11] Dunford RG, Vann RD, Gerth WA, et al. The incidence of venous gas emboli in recreational diving. Undersea Hyperb Med 2002;29(4):247–59.

[12] Marroni A, Bennet P, Cronjé F, et al. A deep stop during decompression from 25 m significantly reduces bubbles and fast tissue gastensions. Undersea Hyperb Med 2004;31(2):233–43.

[13] Gardette B. Correlation between decompression sickness and circulating bubbles in 232 divers. Undersea Biomed Res 1979;6(1):99–107.

[14] Cohnheim J. Trombose und embolie. In: Vorlesungen ueber allgemeine pathologie. Berlin: Hirschwald; 1877. p. 134.

[15] Gronert GA, Messick JM Jr, Cucchiara RF, et al. Paradoxical air embolism from a patent foramen ovale. Anesthesiology 1979;50(6):548–9.

[16] Moon RE, Camporesi EM, Kisslo JA. Patent foramen ovale and decompression sickness in divers. Lancet 1989;1(8637):513–4.

[17] Hagberg M, Ornhagen H. Incidence and risk factors for symptoms of decompression sickness among male and female dive masters and instructors–a retrospective cohort study. Undersea Hyperb Med 2003;30(2):93–102.

[18] Reul J, Weis J, Jung A, et al. Central nervous system lesions and cervical disc herniations in amateur divers. Lancet 1995;345(8962):1403–5.

[19] Arnold-Chiari malformation. DAN Europe Medical FAQ, DAN Europe. Available at: http://www.daneurope.org/eng/faQ.8.htm. Accessed November 1, 2004.

[20] Fisher DC, Fisher EA, Budd JH, et al. The incidence of patent foramen ovale in 1,000 consecutive patients. A contrast transesophageal echocardiography study. Chest 1995;107(6):1504–9.

[21] Job FP, Ringelstein EB, Grafen Y, et al. Comparison of transcranial contrast Doppler sonography and transesophageal contrast echocardiography for the detection of patent foramen ovale in young stroke patients. Am J Cardiol 1994;74(4):381–4.

[22] Hagen PT, Scholz DG, Edwards WD. Incidence and size of patent foramen ovale during the first 10 decades of life: an autopsy study of 965 normal hearts. Mayo Clin Proc 1984;59(1):17–20.

[23] Patten BM. The closure of the foramen ovale. Am J Anat 1931;48:19–44.

[24] Di Tullio M, Sacco RL, Venketasubramanian N, et al. Comparison of diagnostic techniques for the detection of a patent foramen ovale in stroke patients. Stroke 1993;24(7):1020–4.

[25] Germonpre P, Dendale P, Unger P, et al. Patent foramen ovale and decompression sickness in sports divers. J Appl Physiol 1998;84(5):1622–6.

[26] Balestra C, Germonpré P, Snoeck T, et al. PFO detection in divers—methodological aspects. European Journal of Underwater and Hyperbaric Medicine 2002;3(3):74.

[27] Knauth M, Ries S, Pohimann S, et al. Cohort study of multiple brain lesions in sport divers: role of a patent foramen ovale. BMJ 1997;314(7082):701–5.

[28] Tetzlaff K, Friege L, Hutzelmann A, et al. Magnetic resonance signal abnormalities and neuropsychological deficits in elderly compressed-air divers. Eur Neurol 1999;42(4):194–9.

[29] Vermeer SE, Prins ND, den Heijer T, et al. Silent brain infarcts and the risk of dementia and cognitive decline. N Engl J Med 2003;348(13):1215–22.

[30] Balestra C, Marroni A, Farkas B, et al. The fractal approach as a tool to understand asymptomatic brain hyperintense MRI signals. Fractals 2004;12(1):67–72.

[31] Cambier BA, Missault LH, Kockx MM, et al. Influence of the breathing mode on the time course and amplitude of the cyclic inter-atrial pressure reversal in postoperative coronary bypass surgery patients. Eur Heart J 1993;14(7):920–4.

[32] Schneider B, Hofmann T, Justen MH, Meinertz T. Chiari's network: normal anatomic variant or risk factor for arterial embolic events? J Am Coll Cardiol 1995;26(1):203–10.

[33] Vik A, Jenssen BM, Eftedal O, et al. Relationship between venous bubbles and hemodynamic responses after decompression in pigs. Undersea Hyperb Med 1993;20(3):233–48.

[34] Balestra C, Germonpre P, Marroni A. Intrathoracic pressure changes after Valsalva strain and other maneuvers: implications for divers with patent foramen ovale. Undersea Hyperb Med 1998;25(3):171–4.

[35] Ries S, Knauth M, Kern R, et al. Arterial gas embolism after decompression: correlation with right-to-left shunting. Neurology 1999;52(2):401–4.

[36] Cantais E, Louge P, Suppini A, et al. Right-to-left shunt and risk of decompression illness with cochleovestibular and cerebral symptoms in divers: case control study in 101 consecutive dive accidents. Crit Care Med 2003;31(1):84–8.

[37] Germonpre P, Dendaele P, Unger P, et al. Patent foramen ovale in sports diving, a risk factor for certain forms of decompression illness. Acta Cardiologica 1996;51(1):44–5.

[38] Klingmann C, Benton PJ, Ringleb PA, et al. Embolic inner ear decompression illness: correlation with a right-to-left shunt. Laryngoscope 2003; 113(8):1356–61.

[39] Wilmshurst P, Davidson C, O'Connell G, et al. Role of cardiorespiratory abnormalities, smoking and dive characteristics in the manifestations of neurological decompression illness. Clin Sci (Lond) 1994; 86(3):297–303.

[40] Germonpre P. Le foramen oval perméable dans l'accident neurologique de décompression. Revue de la littérature. Bulletin de Medecine Hyperbare et Subaquatigue 1999;9:111–6.

[41] Wilmshurst PT, Pearson MJ, Walsh KP, et al. Relationship between right-to-left shunts and cutaneous decompression illness. Clin Sci (Lond) 2001;100(5): 539–42.

[42] Conkin J, Pilmanis AA, Webb JT. Case descriptions and observations about cutis marmorata from hypobaric decompressions. Report no. TP-2002–210779. Houston (TX): NASA Technical Information Service; 2002.

[43] Rook A, Wilkinson DS, Ebling FJG. Textbook of dermatology. 5th edition. Oxford (UK): Blackwell Scientific Publications; 1992.

[44] Hurwitz S. Cutaneous disorders of the newborn. In: Hurwitz S, editor. Clinical pediatric dermatology: a textbook of skin disorders of childhood and adolescence. 2nd edition. Philadelphia: WB Saunders; 1993. p. 7–39.

[45] Hennessy TR, Hempleman HV. An examination of the critical released gas volume concept in decompression sickness. Proc R Soc Lond B Biol Sci 1977;197(1128):299–313.

[46] Schuknecht HF. Pathology of the ear. Cambridge (MA): Harvard University Press; 1974.

[47] Marroni A. Recreational diving accidents in Europe: DAN Europe report 1994–1995. In: Oriani G, Wattel F, editors. Proceedings of the Twelfth International Congress on Hyperbaric Medicine. Milan (Italy): Best Publishing Company; 1996. p. 623–32.

[48] Cumming B. NDC diving incidents report: British Sub-Aqua Club: Cheshire, United Kingdom; 2002.

[49] Bove AA. Risk of decompression sickness with patent foramen ovale. Undersea Hyperb Med 1998; 25(3):175–8.

[50] Wendling J, Balestra C, Germonpre P. Is screening for foramen ovale feasible? SPUMS J 2001;31(2): 85–9.

[51] Klingmann C, Knauth M, Ries S, et al. Recurrent inner ear decompression sickness associated with a patent foramen ovale. Arch Otolaryngol Head Neck Surg 2002;128(5):586–8.

[52] Van Camp G, Franken P, Melis P, et al. Comparison of transthoracic echocardiography with second harmonic imaging with transesophageal echocardiography in the detection of right to left shunts. Am J Cardiol 2000;86(11):1284–7, A9.

[53] Germonpre P, Balestra C, Masay L, et al. Correlation between patent foramen ovale, MRI cerebral lesions and neuropsychometric testing in experienced sports divers: does diving damage the brain? In: Hyldegaard O, Jansen E, Risby-Mortensen C, editors. Proceedings of the Annual Meeting of the European Underwater and Baromedical Society, 2003. Copenhagen: 2003.

[54] Marabotti C, Chiesa F, Scalzini A, et al. Cardiac and humoral changes induced by recreational scuba diving. Undersea Hyperb Med 1999;26(3):151–8.

[55] Evers S, Altenmuller E, Ringelstein EB. Cerebrovascular ischemic events in wind instrument players. Neurology 2000;55(6):865–7.

[56] Germonpre P, Balestra C, Farkas B, et al. Impact of a newly identified medical condition upon fitness-to-dive criteria: patent foramen ovale—a contra-indication that is not? In: Wendling J, editor. Proceedings of the 6th Consensus Conference of European Committee on Hyperbaric Medicine (ECHM) on Prevention of Diving Accidents. Geneva: ECHM; 2003.

[57] Wilmshurst PT, Byrne JC, Webb-Peploe MM. Relation between interatrial shunts and decompression sickness in divers. Lancet 1989;2(8675):1302–6.

[58] Kerut EK, Truax WD, Borreson TE, et al. Detection of right to left shunts in decompression sickness in divers. Am J Cardiol 1997;79(3):377–8.

[59] Torti SR, Billinger M, Schwerzmann M, et al. Risk of decompression illness among 230 divers in relation to the presence and size of patent foramen ovale. Eur Heart J 2004;25(12):1014–20.

[60] Germonpre P, Balestra C, Unger P, et al. Time-related opening of the foramen ovale in divers. In: Germonpre P, Balestra C, editors. Proceedings of the 28th Annual Meeting of the European Underwater and Baromedical Society, 2002. Bruges (Belgium): Advisory Committee for Hyperbaric Oxygen; 2002.

ELSEVIER
SAUNDERS

Cardiol Clin 23 (2005) 105–107

CARDIOLOGY CLINICS

Index

Note: Page numbers of article titles are in **boldface** type.

Changing Your Address?

Make sure your subscription changes too! When you notify us of your new address, you can help make our job easier by including an exact copy of your Clinics label number with your old address (see illustration below.) This number identifies you to our computer system and will speed the processing of your address change. Please be sure this label number accompanies your old address and your corrected address—you can send an old Clinics label with your number on it or just copy it exactly and send it to the address listed below.

We appreciate your help in our attempt to give you continuous coverage. Thank you.

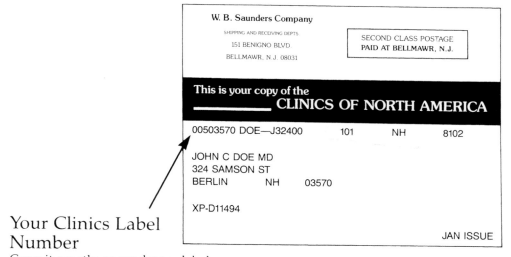

Your Clinics Label Number
Copy it exactly or send your label
along with your address to:
W.B. Saunders Company, Customer Service
Orlando, FL 32887-4800
Call Toll Free 1-800-654-2452

Please allow four to six weeks for delivery of new subscriptions and for processing address changes.